THE BODY SCULPTING BIBLE

EXPRESS

MEN'S EDITION

THE BODY SCULPTING BIBLE

EXPRESS

James Villepigue

Hugo Rivera

Photography by:
Peter Field Peck

healthyliving**books**

New York • London

www.bodysculptingbible.com

MEN'S EDITION

Published by Hatherleigh Press
5-22 46th Avenue, Suite 200
Long Island City, NY 11101
www.hatherleighpress.com

Villepigue, James C.
The body sculpting bible express workout for men : featuring the 21-minute body sculpting workout / by James Villepigue, Hugo Rivera.
p. cm.
ISBN 1-57826-294-6
1. Bodybuilding. 2. Exercise for men. I. Rivera, Hugo A., 1974- II. Title.
GV546.5.V53 2004
613.7'13--dc22
2004021943

ISBN 1-57826-294-6

Disclaimer
All forms of exercise pose some inherent risks. The information in this book is meant to supplement, not replace, proper exercise training. Before practicing the exercises in this book, be sure that your equipment is well-maintained. Do not take risks beyond your level of experience, training, and fitness. The exercise and dietary programs in this book are not intended as a substitute for any exercise routine or treatment or dietary regimen that may have been prescribed by your doctor. As with all exercise and dietary programs, you should get your doctor's approval before beginning. The author, editors, and publisher advise readers to take full responsibility for their safety and know their limits.

THE BODY SCULPTING BIBLE EXPRESS books are available for bulk purchase, special promotions, and premiums. For information on reselling and special purchase opportunities, please call us at 1-800-528-2550 and ask for the Special Sales Manager.

Special thanks to Marie-Annick Courtier, RoseMarie Alfieri and Paul Frediani.

Interior design by Deborah Miller and Calvin Lyte
Cover design by Deborah Miller and Calvin Lyte

10 9 8 7 6 5 4 3 2 1
Printed in United States

Dedication

I would like to dedicate this exciting project to the most important people in my life. To my remarkable mom, Nancy, I am truly blessed by God to be your son and I simply adore you; to my talented sister, Debbie, my love for you could never cease and I am, as I have always said, "So very proud of you!"; to my awesome dad, Jim, I love you always and I miss you so much, pal. I honor you every moment of my life. To God, thank you, thank you, thank you! To Heather, thank you for your incredible support, I love you; to all of my beautiful family and friends, you know who you are and I love you all! Finally, to those of you reading, thank you so much. We hope you enjoy *Express For Men*. Good luck and God bless!

Additionally, I would like to thank the following people: Andrew Flach and Kevin Moran, you have both become dear friends; a heartfelt thank you for all of the wonderful opportunities you have given me. Thank you, Paul Frediani, you are a class act man! To my bro, Peter Field Peck, as always, great work! To RoseMarie Alfieri, you are so awesome! To all of the Hatherleigh Press team, you are all the very best!

James Villepigue

This book is dedicated to my beautiful wife Lina, who always loves and supports me unconditionally throughout any project; to my son Chad, who is my pride and joy; to my parents and grandparents for always believing in me and who always ensured that I would get the best education possible as I grew up; to my brother Raul whose computer knowledge made it possible for me to go online; to my in-laws who are always there to help me and provide me with support in time of need; to William Kemp for being such an awesome mentor and friend; to Chris Lind for all his website help and friendship; and finally to God for giving me the talent to put this work together.

Additionally, special thanks go out to Tim Gardner and Todd Mendelsohn. Without your help, I would not be at the level of development that I am today. Thank you so much for your expertise and your great friendship! Andre Hudson, for being such an inspirational success story, an awesome trainer, and a great friend. Laree Draper, for always being there to offer a hand and for the incredible job you do maintaining Irononline, the best weight training email group in the Internet. Dave Draper, for always leading by example and for being an inspiration to all who follow the body sculpting lifestyle. The people at Prolab Inc., for giving me the opportunity to get more involved in the fitness industry and for putting out such awesome high quality products at a great price. To RoseMarie Alfieri, for your valuable input and awesome help. Last but not least, Andrew Flach and Kevin Moran. Thank you for giving me the opportunity to spread the fitness word to millions of people.

Hugo A. Rivera

Precautions

You should always consult a physician before starting any weight gain or fat reduction training/nutrition program.

A basic metabolic test, thyroid, lipid, and testosterone panel is recommended prior to starting this program in order to detect anything that can prevent you from making the most out of your efforts.

Consult your doctor regarding these tests.

If you are unfamiliar with any of the exercises, consult an experienced trainer to instruct you on the proper form and execution of the unfamiliar exercise. Improper form can lead to injury.

The instructions and advice presented herein are not intended as a substitute for medical or other personal professional counseling.

HR Fitness Inc., the editors, and the authors disclaim any liability or loss in connection with the use of this system, its programs, and advice herein.

Table of Contents

Introduction
Is This Workout for You?

"I have so much free time I don't know what to do with it!" Have you ever heard anyone you know say this—and actually mean it? Chances are the opposite is true. You're more accustomed to hearing and thinking: "How on earth am I going to do everything I need to do? There's just not enough time." Not enough time to get work done, to enjoy ourselves, to be with our friends and our families. Certainly not enough time to exercise!

That's why the *Body Sculpting Bible EXPRESS* workout—a workout you can do in 21 minutes—was created. This is a workout so efficient, it was designed specifically to help you achieve the greatest fitness gains in the least amount of time possible. You may not have enough time to commit to hour-long workouts at a gym a few days a week. But surely you can spare 21 minutes three or four days each week.

THE BODY SCULPTING BIBLE EXPRESS

By now we all know how important it is to incorporate exercise into our lives. Study after study, most particularly the 1996 Report by the Surgeon General of the United States, reveals that people who exercise are healthier and that physical activity helps to improve our outlook on life. Many of us simply want to look better—to have bodies that are strong and cut. In other words, you must find the time to work out.

IS THIS WORKOUT FOR YOU?

Maybe you are an extremely busy guy whose calendar has few blank spaces; perhaps you are raising a family, and devote most of your time and energy to your kids; maybe you are someone who simply does not want to spend your evenings working out, even if you have the time; or maybe you want to get in and get out, and onto other things you enjoy in life. If you fit any of these descriptions, then the 21-Minute *EXPRESS* Workout is for you.

Can you really work out for only 21 minutes and get results? Absolutely. Weight training is a little bit different than other sports. Some, like football and baseball, have complicated playing rules and last a long time, while others, like track and field, are more straight forward; less complicated, quicker, but just as challenging. We often hear men say that they don't feel that it's worth it to go to the gym if they can't do a long, drawn-out workout. In reality, some people spend hours at the gym in a very inefficient way (resting too long between exercises, talking away half their workout, performing too many repetitions, or using weight that is way too light).

While they may be at the gym for an hour plus, they are in fact only benefiting from a fraction of that hour. The essential factor in workouts is a proper structure that efficiently puts exercise science to work for you.

We've designed a program that covers the major muscles in your upper and lower body. In the 21-Minute *EXPRESS* Workout, you move quickly from one exercise to the other, which enables your heart rate to rise into the training zone to get cardiovascular as well as strength and muscle building benefits. We spell out every step of the workout, so that you know what to do, how to do it, and in what order.

You can use the 21-Minute *EXPRESS* Workout in a number of ways. It can be your main workout, or it can complement longer workouts or cardio-only workouts such as running and biking. You can make this the workout you do on those days or weeks when you are pressed for time. It's a great workout to do when traveling as you just need a couple sets of weights. And it's wonderfully suited for people who are just beginning an exercise program, and who want to get good results quickly.

THE 21-DAY CHALLENGE

You will be successful in sculpting your body and enhancing your health and fitness if you make the commitment. In just 21 days, you'll see changes in your body, in the way that you feel, and even the way you think.

That is our challenge to you. Spend 21 minutes a day for 21 days with us, and commit to a higher level of fitness. If you are looking for a jumpstart back into an old routine, this can get you started. If you are looking for a quick set of exercises to keep you fit for life, this is it.

If you're ready to feel stronger, and to know that you are investing in your health and fitness, it's time to take the 21-Day Challenge. At the end, there's nothing that will make you feel better than to look back on your accomplishments.

HOW TO USE THIS BOOK

This book begins with a discussion of the principles of the *EXPRESS* Workout—how and why it works. You'll see that while the workout is short on time, it is long on intensity and this makes all the difference. You'll learn the supporting evidence for this type of workout. We will also present a general protocol for strength training, discussing how to properly lift weights to maximize benefits and minimize risk of injury, and how to set workout goals.

In Chapter 2, we present a general eating plan that supports healthy, active living. You really are what you eat, and you need to make the food choices that will give you the most nutritional bang for the caloric buck. This is especially true when you are exercising and need your body to be full of energy!

Part II presents the exercises that are in the 21-Minute Workout programs. In Chapter 3, we go over the importance of warming up and stretching—a vital, often overlooked, component of any fitness program. You'll find challenging, effective exercises for your back and chest, shoulders and arms, abs, legs, and glutes, as well as a section on combination exercises, which work the lower and upper body at the same time. We've also given you alternative exercises you can do on stack machines if you prefer.

Finally, Part III contains the 21-Day Challenge and your six-week, 21-Minute Workout program featuring workouts that you can perform with just a pair of dumbbells and a bench. Optional workouts are included for stack machines at the gym. While machine workouts are good, you'll get the most out of dumbbell workouts. We will explain this in the next chapter.

SUCCESS DEFINED

In the *Body Sculpting Bible*, we talked about what success is. It's worth reiterating here: success depends on desire, determination, and action. You must want to be successful, and want it strongly. You must be determined to overcome any obstacles you may have (often when it comes to exercise, these are psychological) and, finally, you must actually get up and engage in exercise. You must act. If you have these three qualities, the workouts in this book will help you to obtain a sleeker, leaner body. This can be done in just 21 minutes a session—barely any time at all.

Part I
The Principles of the *EXPRESS* Workout

This part will introduce you to the principle of periodization, a method of training that is scientifically proven to give you the best results. We will also give you all the tools you need to maximize your benefits and minimize your risks, including protocols on the proper way to lift weights, meal plans to support your fitness goals, and tips on how to maintain your motivation.

Chapter 1

21 Minutes to Fitness

THE 21-MINUTE SOLUTION; HOW AND WHY IT WORKS

The Body Sculpting Bible *EXPRESS* Workout was created to provide an efficient workout for those of you who do not have more than 30 minutes a day free to dedicate to fitness. For example, we spoke to many school teachers who have a lot of time during the summer, but when school starts, their workout time gets drastically reduced. This is for people like them.

Now, the question is raised: "Is 21 minutes enough time to get results?" The answer is an emphatic yes! We have to remember that, unlike most things in life, working out more and more reaches a point of diminishing returns. Many times, people who are overly enthusiastic and who exercise too much begin storing body fat and losing muscle. The reason for this is a stress hormone released by the adrenal glands called cortisol. This

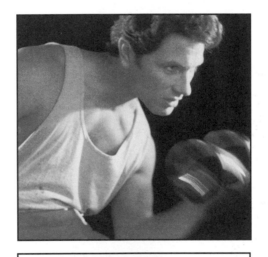

THE BODY SCULPTING BIBLE EXPRESS

1

hormone is affected by exercise, and while its release can be minimized if workouts are kept short, it is released in large quanities when you work out excessively. When it comes to fitness there is only one thing that you need to remember: intensity. If you focus and work hard during the time you are able to work out, you will accomplish more than the people who spend two hours in the gym talking most of the time.

While the workouts from the original *Body Sculpting Bibles* will provide more rapid results, the *EXPRESS* Workouts will provide comparable results in even less time at the gym. In other words, what you could accomplish during six weeks of using the longer workouts, you will be able to accomplish within roughly 10 weeks of using the shorter workouts. Not bad considering that the time invested is minimal.

SUPPORTING SCIENTIFIC EVIDENCE

A study performed in 2002 by researchers from the University of Minnesota and the Mayo Clinic showed that two short 30-minute sessions a week in the gym is all that adults need to experience effective body fat loss and valuable gains in muscle strength and lean muscle mass (*International Journal of Obesity* 27:326-332, 2002). 60 women ranging from ages 30 to 50 years old lost an average of two pounds of fat and gained an average of two pounds of muscle in 15 weeks. There was no monitoring of the participants' diets during the study, so we can assume that there was little or no change of eating habits. Also, the workout rou-

tine the participants used may not have been as effective as it could have been. Remember that men have much more testosterone than women do, so if men had been in the study, the results would have been that much better.

By using the three periodized 21-minute workouts described in this book, coupled with the fat-burning muscle-building dict presented in Chapter 2, you will lose body fat and gain muscle at the fastest rate possible. It is quality, not quantity, that counts the most in the world of fitness.

GOAL SETTING AND THE 21-DAY CHALLENGE

Without goals we are a ship adrift in the middle of the sea. We go with the flow and if we ever get anywhere it is by mere accident. In order to achieve success, we need to clearly define and ingrain our goals in our minds. Otherwise, like the drifting boat, if we get anywhere it will be by mere chance.

This book's goals are designed around the 21-Day Challenge. If you can exercise for 21 minutes a day, every day, for 21 days, you will be well on your way towards getting fit! This workout can be used if you're just beginning and need a starting program for your fitness regime, or if you're returning to the gym after a long absence. This workout lasts for only three weeks, obviously a short-term goal. It's up to you where you want your body to be in the long term.

Do you want to bodybuild, lose inches, or increase your endurance? Decide now, before you even lift a weight. As a small exercise, take out a piece of paper and write down two things. The first will be your long-term goals. Be specific! Write the measurements that you will have (Chest, Arms, Thighs, Calves, and Waist), your body fat percentage and your total body weight. Don't limit yourself to what you think you can achieve; write down what you want. (At the same time, if you are a male body-builder and you want 28-inch arms, know that such a goal is unrealistic. Shoot for 18 to 20 inches instead.) Did you write down your long-term goals? If not, stop reading and do so now!

If you are reading this paragraph we will assume that you wrote down your long-term goals. Now, the problem is that such goals seem so far away. Since every long trip starts with the first step, write down your short-term goals. For the purposes of this *EXPRESS* Workout, the first three weeks will be jumpstarting your fitness regime. It's the second three weeks which will determine your eventual path. Short-term goals should be analyzed every six weeks. Obviously, your short-term goals will be smaller than long-term goals. By having more and more short-term goals, your long-term goals are achievable.   When you write down your goals, be positive and have no doubt in your mind that you can achieve them. This is crucial! So go ahead and write your short-term goals down now. Here's the format:

For the next six weeks I will:		
Lose	_____	pounds of fat
Gain	_____	pounds of muscle
Weigh	_____	pounds
Have measurements of:		
Chest	_____	inches
Arms	_____	inches
Thighs	_____	inches
Calves	_____	inches
Waist	_____	inches

Once you have all of those goals written down, write down what ACTIONS will you take for the next six weeks to get there. For instance:

ACTION PLAN

- I will carry healthy snacks with me to eat between balanced meals

- I will wake up and do cardio first thing in the morning three times a week

- I will do three 21-minute weight-training sessions a week

- I will get a full night of sleep

- I will drink one gallon of water a day

- I will only have one cheat day a week

You can also take pictures of how you currently look (be sure to also document current measurements: body weight, body fat, etc.). This is a great way to stay motivated—when you look at your current pictures, and compare them with pictures of yourself a year later, you will see a huge difference!

Now that you have written all of this down, it is time to move from words to actions. If you follow your action plan religiously and you only miss your goals by a bit, don't get discouraged! You should see progress and this is what we are shooting for; constant progress that will lead us to our ultimate goals.

If you missed your mark because you did not follow your action plan, don't punish yourself. Simply set new goals and be more determined to follow your action plan.

If you mess up your plan for a day, don't drop the whole thing and quit! If you encounter one of these days, begin your recovery the following day by starting the plan again.

Now that you have your goals, we'll talk about the formula for success. After that, we'll present you with an exercise workout that works so that you can go ahead and achieve your plan; the 21-Minute Body Sculpting Bible *EXPRESS* Workout.

THE FORMULA FOR SUCCESS

No matter what your goals are, the formula for success will guarantee that you get the results you want. The only thing that differs is the way in which each individual implements it, because each individual has different goals.

For example, most women like to tone up their waist, legs, and arms while most men are interested in getting large amounts of muscle size everywhere.

The formula is the following:

$$S = D \times (T+N+R)$$

S is the success that you achieve in your program, **D** is the determination that you have to achieve success, **T** is the training that you use, **N** is your nutritional program and **R** stands for rest.

Each component in the formula can be assigned a 0 or a 1. A 1 is given to a component if it is followed completely, and a 0 is given to any component not completed or halfway followed. If every single component is followed, you can get a maximum value of 3. This person will get the fastest results possible from their program. If the person stops training, resting, or eating properly, she will get a smaller value and less than optimal results. However, if you don't have determination, your value is 0 and you won't get any results. Determination is by far the most important factor in your success with your exercise program.

It is now easy to see why purchasing a sophisticated gadget or a couple of magic pills at the health food store is not going to cut it. To achieve permanent results, all of the factors have to be present and in harmony. Follow one but not the other and your success will be negatively affected. Now that you have an idea of what it will take to get the body of your dreams, let's go into each of the individual components of the formula for success.

DETERMINATION

This is the most important by far. If you are not determined enough to make the sacrifices necessary to get in shape, then it's not going to happen. Take the case of one of us (Hugo): *Most people usually think that I have all the time in the world to work out (by the way, most people's excuse for not being in shape is lack of time). When I tell them that I am married, I have a child, and work full time on my business (around 50-60 hours per week) they can't believe it. I can certainly understand that we live in a very busy age. However, please don't tell me that you don't have at least 21 minutes 3 times a week that you can spare to take care of yourself; that is simply unbelievable.* Be determined and stick to your goal!

TRAINING

There are two types of training:

ANAEROBIC WORK (i.e. weight training) is the #1 way to sculpt your body. Why? Weight training is far superior to any other type of exercise because it increases your metabolism, which in turn helps you burn fat, and gives shape to your body.

AEROBIC WORK (i.e. walking) in your Fat Burning Zone (you can calculate your fat burning heart rate with the following formula: (220 – your age) x 0.75) is a good way to accelerate the fat-burning process. You should not overdo it, and this should be used only in addition to a good weight-training pro-

gram. Aerobics should never be used as a substitute for weight training.

NUTRITION

Nutrition and training go hand-in-hand. Have you ever heard people say that as long as you work out you can eat anything you want because the workout will burn it off? That is wrong! You cannot go every day to McDonalds and get a Big Mac with fries.

If you follow the wrong diet, or follow no eating plan at all, rest assured that your training efforts will be sabotaged and you will have no results at all.

REST AND RECOVERY

You need seven to nine hours of sleep each night for your body to run efficiently. Deprive your body of sleep and your fat loss will suffer. You'll lose muscle, which in turn will lower your metabolism. You'll also deprive your hormonal production, which makes it difficult to build muscle. Finally, there is research that points to the fact that sleep deprivation may be linked to the following:

1. Heart disease
2. Depression
3. Bad temper
4. Lack of concentration and lethargy

Make sure that you get your ZZZ's or else your body will not be operating at peak efficiency.

STRUCTURE AND PRINCIPLES OF THE WORKOUT; WHY AND HOW IT WORKS.

The workout was structured to allow for three days of weights and three days of abdominals.

The abdominal workout can be done in the comfort of your home at any time and will take you approximately six minutes to complete. For faster fat-burning results, you can perform an optional vigorous 15-minute session of cardiovascular activity.

The weight workout splits the body into two parts:

DAY 1: Chest, Back, Biceps, Triceps

DAY 2: Shoulders, Thighs, Hamstrings, Calves

DAY 3: Full Body Workout

This split emphasizes balance in the physique as all major muscle groups are stimulated. A lot of guys suffer from "chest and arms syndrome," where these body parts are the only ones worked out. This leads to an incomplete physique, and also to muscle strength imbalances that can result in injuries. Many men feel that their legs do not need any work. This is wrong. If you fail to train your legs, you will look like a light bulb with two toothpicks on the bottom, and you will miss out on extra upper body growth brought about by the increased hormonal levels due to weight training your legs. Research indicates that exercises like squats and deadlifts bring about the largest hormonal response (increases in testosterone and growth hormone) because virtually all muscles of the body are used in one way or another.

The *EXPRESS* Workout uses free weights (dumbbells) and the 14-Day Body Sculpting Principles to create the fastest results. The program is based on your body's physiology. It usually takes your body 14 days to get used to a new practice, whether that practice is following a diet, a new exercise program, or just getting up earlier in the morning. Getting used to a new practice, such as waking up early to exercise, is a great thing. However, getting used to an exercise program is not as great. Why? Once your body gets used to it, it will stop responding and your results (i.e. fat loss and increased muscle tone) will come to a screeching halt. That is why most people who go to the gym experience great results initially, but later see and feel themselves going nowhere. The key to experiencing continued results is variation. However, the variation cannot be haphazard. You must have a plan that will guarantee continual results; such as the Body Sculpting Bible *EXPRESS* Workout.

For the first two weeks you will use modified compound supersets. This means performing one exercise, resting a prescribed amount of time, going to the next exercise, resting the prescribed amount of time, and going to the next until the circuit is done. Once the circuit is completed, you start at the beginning and repeat for the recommended amount of times. During this two-week period of modified superset use, your body gets stronger as rest periods

MONDAY	TUESDAY	WEDNESDAY	THURSDAY	FRIDAY	SATURDAY	SUNDAY
Day 1	Abs/Cardio	Day 2	Abs/Cardio	Day 3	Abs/Cardio	Off
Day 2	Abs/Cardio	Day 1	Abs/Cardio	Day 3	Abs/Cardio	Off

are abundant and repetitions are at a higher range (12-15). Working out this way allows your nervous system to recover and your body to increase its strength. In addition, the high repetitions allow your body to build more capillaries (necessary for the delivery of nutrients to the muscle cell) and prepare the joints for the heavier weights to come. On weeks 3 and 4 you will start supersetting, or performing one exercise after the other without rest for some of the exercises. The workout becomes more intense in nature, thus creating a higher demand on the central nervous system. Heavier weights and fewer reps (10-12) with a slightly higher number of sets are used as well. The increased volume and the shock to the body created by the increased stress of the weight training routine causes an increased output of growth hormone (that greatly enhances fat loss and muscle tone) and an increase in your metabolism. When your body adapts to this routine, you further add to the intensity by increasing the number of sets, using heavier weights (8-10 reps) and Giant Sets performing four exercises, one after the other, without rest. Once again the body is shocked, growth hormone output goes through the roof, and your metabolism is jolted. The routine is so intense that if you were to maintain it for more than two weeks you would enter a state of overtraining (a state where your body cannot recover from the demands imposed by the intense routine). When your body reaches this level, you will give your body a chance to recover for the next couple of weeks by returning to Week 1.

Are you going backwards? Not at all! With this program you are always moving forward. Even though you are going back to a less stressful type of training with less volume, you will notice that you are now stronger on the same exercises that you had previously worked with. You will use greater weights for the 12-15 repetition range because your body naturally built up its nervous system energies to the highest level possible. Now that your exercise is less stressful you'll have all of this extra energy to get even stronger and more muscular. That is how your strength will increase. After two weeks of modified compound supersets, once again you'll begin to increase the stress on your body and continue this results-producing cycle.

Why is it necessary to get strong and why should you lift heavier weights? Building up your strength through progressive resistance training is the key to increased muscle tone and accelerated fat loss. Remember, if your strength stays the same, your body will look the same.

BEGINNERS AND THE EXPRESS WORKOUT

The Body Sculpting Bible *EXPRESS* Workout is designed for guys who have at least six weeks of training experience. If you are a beginner, you need to perform the same routine laid out in the first two weeks of the program for a period of six weeks. It will take your body approximately six weeks to adjust and get used to the movements, and makes this most efficient for recruiting muscle fibers. It will also give your cardiovascular system a chance to get into shape. By the end of the six weeks, you should have lost a significant amount of weight and you should start seeing more muscle tone and definition in your body. You should also be able to reach your target heart rate by the end of this period. Beginners can also jumpstart their fitness program by taking the 21-Day Challenge presented in Chapter 10.

BEST TIME TO WORK OUT

We recommend you work out in the morning as soon as you awake. Drink 16 ounces of cold water before you start the workout and an additional 30 to 60 ounces during the activity. This is essential to prevent dehydration. We recommend working out first thing in the morning on an empty stomach because you will burn 300 percent more body fat this way. In the morning, your body doesn't have any carbohydrates to burn. In the absence of carbohydrates, your body goes straight to the fat stores in order to get the energy necessary to do the work. Another good reason to work out in the morning is growth hormone levels are at their highest levels (one of the hormones responsible for muscle growth and influencing fat loss). Working out in the morning will allow you to expedite fat loss for dramatic results. However, we do understand that certain obstacles, such as work constraints, might not permit you to train in the morning. In this case, do your cardio or weight training two or three hours after any meal (if your last meal was at 3 p.m., then your exercise session should be at 5 or 6 p.m.).

WORKOUT CLOTHING

Wear comfortable clothes that allow your body to move freely without constraints. Therefore, rigid clothes like jeans and the like are definitely out of the question. You also need to choose clothes based on the climate and environmental conditions. You should wear extra layers of clothing if it is cold to help keep your body temperature warm and prevent possible injuries. Wear comfortable cross training shoes along with a thick absorbent pair of socks. Never train in your bare feet or with sandals; you could seriously injure your feet if you dropped a plate or a dumbbell.

HOW FAST SHOULD YOU LIFT THE WEIGHT?

This fascinating topic is one that many people in the fitness industry have had difficulty agreeing upon. "Should I lift the weight fast? Should I lift the weight slow? Should I move the weight fast or slow on the positive (concentric) portion of the rep? Should I move fast or slow on the negative (eccentric) portion of the rep?" All of these are very good questions and should all be researched. In fact, we have done the research and will now answer each one in detail.

We have found that slow lifting is usually only good for beginners that have never lifted a weight before. It helps them to learn and master the movement and prevents them from using bad exercise form. However, as you become more advanced, science and our own experience indicate that you should lift the weight as quickly as possible without sacrificing form and without involving momentum (jerking and bouncing of the weights). You create more force lifting fast and therefore more muscle fibers are activated. If you do not use momentum to help move the weight, then the force you generate during the movement is created solely by your muscles and not inertia. This is what helps stimulate your muscles to grow, and creates the tone and shape that you so desire. While some might believe that super slow lifting is beneficial because it is difficult to perform and painful, it is not the best way to stimulate muscle growth. Super-slow lifting accumulates too much lactic acid within your muscles and fatigues them before they reach real momentary muscular failure.

Science tells us that Force = Mass (in this case the weight you are lifting) times Acceleration (the increasing speed at which you lift the weight). Therefore, the best way to lift weights is to lift them fast, with total control of the weight and void of momentum. Since you won't be jerking the weights or using ballistic movements during exercise, the risk of getting injured is no greater than the risk of getting injured lifting super slowly.

One last thing about lifting speed: If you are lifting a weight that only allows you to do 8 repetitions, it might look like you are lifting the weight slowly even though you are lifting it as fast as possible. This is due to the fact that the heavier the weight the slower you will be able to move it, even though you are trying to accelerate as fast as you can. This is amazing! We are sure you've heard people's concerns about how lifting heavier weights is dangerous, right? It is actually the opposite. When you lift lighter weights, you have the ability to move the weights very quickly and sloppily because little stress is put upon the muscles, tissues, and joints. This creates a greater risk for injuries to occur. When you lift heavier weights, you are forced to go slower and to use controlled form. Lifting heavier weights will stimulate more muscle fibers while limiting the chance for injury. On the other hand, do not lift a weight if you cannot lift it for a minimum of eight repetitions. Heavier weights may indeed cause connective tissue injury.

HOW TO BREATHE WHILE PERFORMING THE EXERCISE

The correct way to breathe while performing an exercise is to exhale (breathe out) while you are forcing the weight up (the concentric phase a.k.a. muscle contraction) and to inhale (breathe in) while you are lowering or releasing the weight (the eccentric phase a.k.a. the negative portion of the exercise). For example, if you are doing a bench press, you exhale while you push the weight away from your body and inhale while you lower the weight towards your chest.

HOW TO SELECT THE WEIGHT FOR EACH EXERCISE

The weight you select for each exercise depends on the number of repetitions that you need to do for a particular set. If you need to do between 10-12 repetitions for one set, then you need to pick a weight where you fail (the

MUSCLE SORENESS

Muscle soreness is caused by microtrauma to the muscles and is a good indicator that the workout you performed was effective. If you have never exercised before, you will experience higher levels of soreness than usual at the beginning of your program. That is OK. As your body gets used to the exercise program, the muscle soreness will subside to tolerable levels. You just need to persevere through those first few weeks. Do not confuse this type of soreness with overtraining.

There are several degrees of soreness that you need to be aware of:

- Delayed Onset Muscle Soreness
- Typical Mild Muscle Soreness
- Injury-Type Muscle Soreness

The first type of soreness is delayed onset muscle soreness (DOMS). The term DOMS refers to the deep muscular soreness usually experienced two days (not the day after) after the exercise has been done. DOMS prevents the total muscular contraction from occurring within a muscle. This type of severe soreness is caused when you either embark on an exercise program for the first time or when you train a body part harder than usual. It can last for a couple of days for an advanced well-conditioned athlete or for as long as a week for a beginner. If this type of soreness is affecting you and it is time to work out again, the best thing to do is to exercise the affected body part in an active recovery routine. In active recovery routines, all of the loads are reduced by 50 percent, and the sets are not taken to muscular failure. For example, if you are to perform an exercise for 10 repetitions, divide the weight that you usually use for that exercise by two. Stop performing the exercise even though you may not reach muscular failure at the tenth rep. Active recovery helps to restore full movement in the muscle, helping to remove the lactic acid and other waste products building up within the muscles. It also forces high concentrations of blood into the damaged area of the muscles and nourishes the muscles for repair and growth. We find that doing this is always beneficial; by the next day you will not be as sore or stiff as you ordinarily would have been had you skipped a workout to wait for the pain to subside.

The second type of soreness is the typical mild muscle soreness experienced the day after a good workout. While scientists are still unable to pinpoint the true cause of such soreness, the explanation generally accepted is that it is caused by microtrauma at the muscle fiber level and by an excess of lactic acid. At any rate, what's important is that this is a good mild soreness that does not impair muscle function like DOMS. The pain generally lasts a day for advanced athletes and up to three days for a beginner. This soreness, on average, indicates that you had a good workout the day before because you created the trauma necessary to trigger adaptation (e.g. muscle growth). When you are no longer experiencing this type of soreness, it is a good indication that your body has successfully adapted to the training program. This is not one of the goals you will be striving for, as it leads to no gains. And, this is the reason why our program changes on a consistent basis.

The third type of soreness is the one caused by injury. This soreness is entirely different in nature from the ones described above, as it is usually immobilizing and triggers very sharp pain within the muscles and/or joints. Depending on the nature of the injury, the pain might either be experienced constantly or only when the joints are moved or muscles contract. These injuries often become apparent as soon as they happen. Other times they appear either the day after and sometimes days after the activity. If you suddenly become injured, the first thing that you should do is apply the RICE principle (Rest, Ice, Compression, and Elevation). After consulting a doctor, who might allow you to continue training, carefully work around the injury (in other words, utilize exercises that work around the injured muscle(s), without overstepping the range of motion that triggers the pain). More serious injuries, such as a muscle tear, may involve complete rest of the injured and surrounding areas and, depending on the severity, possibly surgery. The best way to prevent this type of injury, pain, and soreness, is by cycling your exercise parameters and by constantly practicing good form.

OVERTRAINING

Overtraining is a condition caused when the body is taxed beyond its ability to recover. The main causes may include long workouts, an overload of training volume (too many sets and reps), a poor diet, lack of sleep, etc. People experiencing this condition might notice such symptoms as a loss of muscle mass, weakness, trouble sleeping, loss of appetite, a lethargic and constant tired feeling, or feelings of depression.

It is impossible to overtrain with our weight-training program (assuming you follow the nutrition and rest practices) because after you stress the body's recuperative capabilities to the maximum (by doing supersets for two weeks and then moving on to Giant Sets for two more), you back off into the less stressful modified compound supersets. In addition, you get a rest day after every day of lifting and the weekends off. During rest days, you concentrate on optional fat burning aerobic exercise (that aids in the recuperation process by removing the lactic acid created by weight training). Sunday is our total inactivity day. This day serves to rest the body and the mind. Finally, the short duration of the workout coupled with ample nutrients provided by the diet, along with the recommended supplements, eliminate the possibility of getting overtrained.

Provided that you follow the training program as laid out, in conjunction with the nutrition and rest components, you should not suffer from overtraining.

point at which completing another repetition becomes impossible) between 10-12 reps. This takes a bit of practice but after a while you will become extremely accurate when it comes to choosing the correct weight for a particular repetition range. If you pick a weight that allows you to do more than 12 repetitions, you'll need to increase the amount of weight being lifted. If you reach failure before hitting the 10th rep, you'll need to decrease the amount of weight. For example, if you are doing four sets of an exercise, as you work through the sets, fatigue will set in and you may not be able to continue using the weight that you chose to lift during the first set. When you get to the point where you can no longer lift a particular weight for a pre-determined repetition range, simply decrease the weight and prepare yourself for the next set.

MISSING WORKOUTS

Missing workouts is unacceptable. You hear it all the time: people making excuses about having no time to exercise. Unless you are on call 24 hours a day, you can find the time to train. If you are interested in completely changing the way you look and feel, all the excuses in the world cannot hold you back from doing what it takes to fit a workout into your schedule. All you need is the vision, the motivation, and the determination to do so.

Missing workouts will severely jeopardize your toning and fat-burning efforts, and destroy your bodysculpter's mindset. If for some reason you are not able to train then make up the missed session the next day. This might mean sacrificing your Sunday rest day or weight-training on abs/optional cardio day, in which case you can either do both workouts at the same time (extending the length of the session to around 45 minutes) or have several sessions that day.

In conclusion, if you miss a workout for whatever reason, don't beat yourself up. Tomorrow is a new day and you will be able to make up the missed session. However, don't make a habit of missing training sessions, as missing sessions will ultimately limit your results.

EQUIPMENT NEEDED

The workout routines in this book use dumbbell-based exercises. Training must consist primarily of free weight exercises in order to bring about the fastest results because these exercises recruit the most muscle. In addition, the body is designed to be in a three-dimensional universe. Whenever you use a machine, you limit your body to a two-dimensional universe and consequently limit the number of muscle fibers doing work.

Not all machines are bad. Some definitely have a place in our weight-training program because they isolate the muscle in a way that no free weights can. However, our program should be based on dumbbell exercises for the reason explained above and also because you can perform this fast moving routine at home or at a crowded gym just by getting some dumbbells and a bench.

MACHINE-BASED ROUTINES FOR VACATION

Typically most hotels do a good job of having weight machines in their fitness rooms but not free weights. Because of this, the book includes a weight machine-only routine that you can use when on vacation. All you have to do is use the routine corresponding to the week that you were on in order to keep from missing workouts. For instance, if you were on weeks 3-4 of the free weights program, then use the machine-based routines presented under those same weeks. While you are not getting as much benefit as you would from a free weight routine, you can still continue your workouts, which is far better than not working out at all.

Chapter 2

Eating for Health and Fitness

In order to make impressive changes to your body, nutrition and training need to go hand in hand. It is a myth that a person can eat as much as they want as long as they exercise. Only people with extremely fast metabolic rates (rate at which the body burns calories) can get away with this. Having said that, with so many diets on the market, we understand why it can be difficult to know what sort of nutrition program is best to follow for the fastest results.

Before covering the diet that we feel is most appropriate based on our personal experiences and clients' results, we'll cover some nutrition basics.

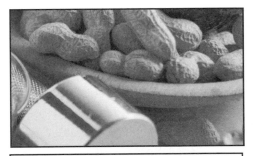

THE BODY SCULPTING BIBLE EXPRESS

2

NUTRITION BASICS

There are three macronutrients that the human body needs in order to function properly.

CARBOHYDRATES

Carbohydrates are your body's main source of energy. When you ingest carbohydrates your pancreas releases a hormone called insulin. Insulin is very important because:

1. It grabs the carbohydrates and either stores them in the muscle or stores them as fat.

2. It grabs the amino acids (protein) and shelters them inside the muscle cell for recovery and repair.

Most overweight people on low fat/high carbohydrate diets eat too many carbohydrates, releasing too much insulin and thus storing fat. There are complex carbohydrates and simple carbohydrates. The complex carbohydrates give you sustained energy ("timed release") while the simple carbohydrates give you immediate energy. You should eat mainly complex carbohydrates throughout the day except for your post-workout meal.

STARCHY COMPLEX CARBOHYDRATES: oatmeal, sweet potatoes, potatoes, rice, grits, or cream of rice.

FIBROUS COMPLEX CARBOHYDRATES: broccoli, carrots, cauliflower, green beans, lettuce, mushrooms, pepper, spinach, or zucchini.

SIMPLE CARBOHYDRATES: apples, bananas, grapefruit, grapes, oranges, pears, pineapple, or peaches.

PROTEIN

Proteins are the building blocks of muscle tissue. Without it, building muscle and burning fat efficiently would be impossible. It increases your metabolism every time you eat it by up to 20 percent, and helps with carbohydrates' timed release.

Everybody involved in a weight-training program should consume between 1 to 1.5 grams of protein per pound of lean body mass (meaning that if you are 100 pounds, and have 10 percent body fat, you should consume at least 90 grams of protein since your lean body mass equals 90 pounds). Nobody should consume more than 1.5 grams per pound of lean body mass as this is unnecessary and the extra protein may get turned into fat.

Good examples of protein are eggs, chicken breast, turkey, 90% lean red meats, and tuna.

FATS

All the cells in your body have some fat in them. Hormones are manufactured from fats. Fats also lubricate your joints. If you eliminate the fat from your diet, your hormonal production will plummet and a whole array of chemical reactions will be interrupted. Your body will then start accumulating more body fat than usual so that it has enough fat to keep on functioning. Since testosterone production is halted, so is muscle building. Therefore, in order to have an efficient metabolism we need fat.

There are three types of fats: saturated, polyunsaturated, and monounsaturated.

SATURATED FATS: Saturated fats are associated with heart disease and high cholesterol levels. They are found to a large extent in products of animal origin. Some vegetable fats also contain large amounts of saturated fats and are generally found in packaged foods. Coconut oil, palm oil, palm kernel oil, and non-dairy creamers are also highly saturated.

POLYUNSATURATED FATS: These fats do not have an effect in cholesterol levels. Most of the fats in vegetable oils, such as canola oil, corn oil, cottonseed, safflower, soybean, and sunflower oil are polyunsaturated. When you consume this fat, it should be from flaxseed oil and fish oils. They are usually high in the essential fatty acids and may have antioxidant properties.

MONOUNSATURATED FATS: These fats have a positive effect on the good cholesterol levels by lowering the bad and increasing the good cholesterol. Sources of these fats are extra virgin olive oil and nuts such as cashews, pecans, and almonds. Peanuts fit in here too although it is really a bean rather than a nut. The main source of your monounsaturated fats should be extra virgin olive oil.

We recommend that 20 percent of your calories come from good fats. Any less than 20% and your hormonal production decreases. Any more than 20% and you start accumulating plenty of fat. Good sources of fat are extra virgin olive oil, natural peanut butter, flaxseed oil, and fish oils.

THE LOW-CARB MYTH

Today the dieting craze is low-carb dieting, where carbohydrates are reduced to 30-50 grams per day in an effort to accelerate weight loss.

So, do these diets work? They do in a way, but not any better than what we call the balanced approach. The key to ensure that the low-carb diets work is to take most of the allotted carbohydrates in the form of vegetables like broccoli and green beans. Your saturated fats are limited to no more than 30 grams per day and most of your fat intake comes from extra virgin olive oil, fish oils, and flaxseed oil. Nuts are good too but they have carbohydrates so you have to be careful with them.

I (Hugo) have used these types of diets for as long as a year with the modifications described above and here are my conclusions:

If you are only allowed 30-50 grams of carbohydrates a day, your life will not be very tasty. You will only be limited to a small selection of foods.

Even though at the beginning you lose incredible amounts of weight, it is mostly water weight. I also did not find a big difference between losing fat in a low-carb diet versus fat on a moderate carbohydrate diet like the one described in the following section.

While on a low-carbohydrate diet, the muscles feel flat (shrink in size) because glycogen (carbohydrates stored inside the muscle cell that make the muscles look firm) is depleted. On a moderate carbohydrate diet, your muscles always feel firm and tight.

DRINK WATER

Water is by far the most abundant substance in our body. Without water, an organism would not survive very long.

- Over 65 percent of your body is composed of water (most of the muscle cell is water).

- Water cleanses your body of toxins and pollutants.

- Water is needed for all of the complex chemical reactions your body performs on a daily basis, such as energy production, muscle building, and fat burning. A lack of water interrupts all of these processes.

- Water helps lubricate the joints.

- When the outside temperature rises, water serves as a coolant to bring the body temperature down.

- Water helps control your appetite. Sometimes when you feel hungry after a good meal this sensation indicates a lack of water. Drinking water at that time would take the craving away.

- Cold water increases your metabolism.

In order to know how much water your body needs a day, just multiply your lean body weight by 0.66. The resulting number indicates how many ounces of water you need in a day.

I experienced joint pains after the ninth month. I was drinking two gallons of water a day, so lack of fluids was not the problem. Once I switched back to a moderate carb diet, the joint pains disappeared.

You have to pay close attention to your cholestcrol levels and to nutritional deficiencies caused by the lack of variety in the diet. In order to get all the good fats in the diet, I had to take them in liquid form—not very tasty.

Even though this diet might work, it will be hard to maintain for a lifetime. As a matter of fact, we see that most people are so restricted on this plan that once they go off, they become compulsive overeaters. While this does not happen to everyone, it does happen. Also, after a few months on the diet, your weight loss plateaus as your thyroid adjusts downward due to the lack of carbohydrates. This in turn lowers your metabolism.

If you feel like trying a low-carb diet, please remember to pay close attention to your cholesterol levels and nutritional deficiencies. Finally, keep in mind that while you can eat slightly more calories on a low-carb plan without storing them as fat, there is a caloric limit after which you will start storing body fat even in the absence of carbs. Therefore, like any diet, remember to create a small caloric deficit.

Having said all this, we believe that to get in shape the best approach is a more balanced diet like the one in the following section.

THE BALANCED APPROACH

In the balanced approach, we use a diet that contains all of the macronutrients in a balanced manner. The breakdown of the nutrient ratios for your diet looks like this:

40% Carbs

40% Protein

20% Fats

CHARACTERISTICS OF A GOOD NUTRITION PROGRAM

YOUR NUTRITION PLAN SHOULD BE BASED ON EATING SMALL AND FREQUENT MEALS THROUGHOUT THE DAY.

When you feed your body several times a day, your metabolism greatly increases. Your body uses food as energy to fuel your metabolism efficiently, burning more fat. If you neglect to feed your body, and wait over three or four hours for consumption, your body switches to a catabolic state and believes it is starving. It begins to feed on your lean muscle tissue, your body's water, your organ tissue, and begins to store your ingested calories as fat for future use. The diet industry has made us think that the key to losing fat is an extreme restriction of calories, but this is not true!

During the Body Sculpting Bible *EXPRESS* program, try to eat between five to six meals a day.

YOUR MEALS SHOULD CONTAIN CARBOHYDRATES, PROTEIN, AND FAT IN THE CORRECT RATIOS.

When you eat a meal that does not contain the proper balance of nutrients (for example, an all carbohydrate meal such as pasta), you will not yield the desired results. Every macronutrient has to be present in order for the body to absorb and use them efficiently. If you only eat carbohydrates, your energy levels will drop in about 30 minutes and unused carbs will be stored as body fat. If you eat only protein, your energy will be low and your body cannot turn protein into lean muscle tissue. The ratios for each particular macronutrient have to be correct to get the results that you desire.

NO SMOKING AND LIMITED ALCOHOL CONSUMPTION.

Both lower testosterone levels (among many other potential problems). Alcohol in particular is greatly responsible for increased fat gain since each gram of alcohol has 7 calories, mostly derived from carbohydrates.

CALORIC REQUIREMENTS

Caloric requirements for most men fluctuate between 2000 and 2500 calories per day. However, if you eat the same number of calories day in and day out, your body will get used to that amount and you will stop losing fat. Therefore, we recommend that you alternate between 2000 and 2500 calories. For two weeks you will consume 2000 calories and then the following two weeks you will consume 2500.

Once you know the total number of calories you need to take in every day, calculate the amount (in grams) of each nutrient by using the percentages above:

Total amount of carbs for the day = (Total number of calories x 0.40)/4

Total amount of protein for the day = (Total number of calories x 0.40)/4

Total amount of fat for the day = (Total number of calories x 0.20)/9

Note: Carbs and protein are divided by five because there are four calories per gram of carbs or of protein. For fats, we divide by nine since there are nine calories for every gram of fat).

2500-CALORIE WEEK MACRONUTRIENT REQUIREMENTS

250 grams of carbohydrates (mostly complex with simple carbs saved for after the workout)
250 grams of protein
55 grams of fats

In six meals that comes out to approximately:
42 grams of carbs per meal
42 grams of protein per meal
9 grams of fats per meal

Dividing all of the results from the formulas above by five (by six if you are eating six times a day) gives you the amount of each nutrient that you will need to consume per meal. As you see, you will be eating between five and six times a day to keep your metabolism high. You don't have to ensure that you get the exact amount that the formula gives you at each and every meal; however, you do have to make sure that you stay within +/- 10 grams of the formula when counting protein and carbs and +/-5 grams when counting fats.

CHOOSING WHAT TO EAT

One of the biggest challenges we face when starting a diet is deciding what to eat every day. Now that you have calculated the amount of carbs, protein, and fats you need for each meal, you need to choose what foods to eat. For this purpose, the food groups table found in Appendix B contains the food values for the foods we recommend you eat should you wish to alter the sample meal plan on the following pages. It is very accurate. However, with so much food processing going on in the food industry these days, it can get tricky. If you happen to discover a discrepancy between the nutritional information on a food label and the chart, believe the food label instead, as we cannot tell what additives they might have decided to add to their ingredients.

Change the times in the Sample Meal Plan to fit your own schedule (we have used the typical 8 a.m.-5 p.m. work day). The post-workout meal assumes that you are training in the morning. If this is not the case, then just have some complex carbs in the morning and move the post-workout meal to the time after your workout is done.

> ## 2000-CALORIE WEEK MACRONUTRIENT REQUIREMENTS
>
> 200 grams of carbohydrates (mostly complex with simple carbs being saved for after the workout)
> 200 grams of protein
> 45 grams of fats
>
> In five meals that comes out to approximately:
> 40 grams of carbs per meal
> 40 grams of protein per meal
> 9 grams of fats per meal

SAMPLE MENU

On the following pages, we have given you a complete menu plan that will aid you in constructing your diet. Remember to have lower calories for two weeks and higher for the following two! If you would like to adapt this menu to your own schedule and liking, please see Appendix B for instructions and food charts.

STRIVE FOR CONSISTENCY INSTEAD OF ABSOLUTE PERFECTION

Many times we see dieters that start out doing great. However, there comes a day that for some reason they miss a workout or they blow their diets. After that day, they become so discouraged that they continue missing workouts or destroy their diets with self-sabotage. Many weeks go by before they get back on track (if ever). In the meantime, muscle tone fades and fat pounds pile up. Please remember the following: we are all human and we are entitled to make mistakes. Always strive for perfection, but if for some reason things don't go as well as they should on a given day, pick up and move on. Jump right back into your program. If you blow a meal one day, don't make it any worse by eating incorrectly all day long. If you miss a workout, don't wait until next Monday to start over. Just continue with your program the way it is laid out. In the end it will be your determination and consistency that will enable you to win the battle of the bulge.

TROUBLESHOOTING YOUR CALORIC INTAKE

The optimum fat loss per week is two pounds. Any more than two pounds a week and you will lose muscle, which will result in the loss of muscle tone, which yields a saggy look and a significantly lower metabolism. Having said that, we need to point out that while most men burn between 2000 to 2500 calories, some have a higher metabolism. Therefore, some men may find themselves losing more than two pounds a week at the prescribed number of calories and others may find themselves gaining weight. If this is the case, don't panic! If you find you are losing too much, simply add 300 calories to both the lower calorie diet and the higher calorie diet. Your diet will fluctuate between 2300 and 2800 calories. After two weeks you should assess how this is working by measuring your lean body mass. If you are still losing weight, again increase calories by an additional 300 and repeat the process until you reach the caloric intake that allows for a two-pound fat loss while at the same time adds muscle tone.

The reverse applies if you are suddenly gaining

MENU PLAN FOR LOW CALORIE WEEKS (2 Week Duration)

Meal 1   (7:30 AM)

CARB OPTIONS:

    3/4 cup of dry oats mixed with water   -or-

    5 tablespoons of Farina (measured dry)   -or-

    1/4 cup of cream of rice (measured dry)   -or-

    1/2 cup of grits (measured dry)

SIMPLE CARBS (assuming this is a post workout meal; otherwise switch this with the meal that falls after your workout):

    1 large banana

PROTEIN OPTIONS:

    3/4 cup of Egg Beaters (measured uncooked)   -or-

    1 1/2 scoop of whey protein (approximately 30-35 grams of protein)

Meal 2   (10:30 AM)

PROTEIN SHAKE:

    Meal replacement shake such as Prolab's Naturally Lean Matrix   -or-

    1 scoop of protein powder such as Prolab's Protein Component mixed with 16 ounces of skim milk

GOOD FATS:

    1 teaspoon of flaxseed oil

Meal 3   (12:30 PM)

CARB OPTIONS:

    3/4 cup of brown or white rice   -or-

    small sized baked potato   -or-

    small sized sweet potato   -or-

    3/4 cup of oatmeal (measured dry)

VEGETABLE OPTIONS (Fibrous Carbs):

    2 cups of green beans mixed with any other desired vegetable   -or-

    2 cups of broccoli mixed with any other desired vegetable

PROTEIN OPTIONS:

    6 ounces of chicken   -or-

    6 ounces of turkey   -or-

    6 ounces of lean fish such as tuna, grouper, red snapper   -or-

    6 ounces of 97% lean steak such as top round sirloin

Meal 4   (3:30 PM)

PROTEIN SHAKE:

    Meal replacement shake such as Prolab's Naturally Lean Matrix -or-

    1 scoop of protein powder such as Prolab's Protein Component mixed with 16 ounces of skim milk

GOOD FATS:

    1 teaspoon of flaxseed oil

Meal 5   (6:30 PM)

CARB OPTIONS:

    3/4 cup of brown or white rice   -or-

    small sized baked potato   -or-

    small sized sweet potato   -or-

    3/4 cup of oatmeal (measured dry)

VEGETABLE OPTIONS (FIBROUS CARBS):

    2 cups of green beans mixed with any other desired vegetable   -or-

    2 cups of broccoli mixed with any other desired vegetable

PROTEIN OPTIONS:

    6 ounces of chicken   -or-

    6 ounces of turkey   -or-

    6 ounces of lean fish such as tuna, grouper, red snapper   -or-

    6 ounces of 97% lean steak such as top round sirloin

Meal 6   (8:30 PM)

CARB OPTIONS:

    You may choose any of the carb options from Meal 1 or 3 but for if fat loss is the main goal then limit carbs to the fibrous choices below:

VEGETABLE OPTIONS (FIBROUS CARBS):

    2 cups of green beans mixed with any other desired vegetable   -or-

    2 cups of broccoli mixed with any other desired vegetable

PROTEIN OPTIONS:

    6 ounces of chicken   -or-

    6 ounces of turkey   -or-

    6 ounces of lean fish such as tuna, grouper, red snapper   -or-

    6 ounces of 97% lean steak such as top round sirloin   -or-

    1 1/2 scoop of protein powder such as Prolab's Protein Component mixed with water

GOOD FATS:

RECOMMENDED SUPPLEMENTS:

MULTIPLE VITAMIN/ MINERAL PAKS:

PROLAB's Training Paks

MEAL REPLACEMENT POWDERS:

PROLAB's Naturally Lean Matrix

PROTEIN POWDERS:

PROLAB's Protein Component

FLAXSEED OIL:

Spectrum's flaxseed oil as it is always kept refrigerated on the way to the retail store.

If following the Advanced Program, the following supplements may also be useful:

CREATINE:

PROLAB's Creatine Monohydrate Powder

GLUTAMINE:

PROLAB's Glutamine Powder

MENU PLAN FOR HIGH CALORIE WEEKS (2 Week Duration)

1 teaspoon of olive oil

Meal 1 (7:30 AM)

CARB OPTIONS:

1 cup of dry oats mixed with water	-or-
6 tablespoons of Farina (measured dry)	-or-
1/3 cup of cream of rice (measured dry)	-or-
1 cup of grits (measured dry)	

SIMPLE CARBS (assuming this is a post workout meal; otherwise switch this with the meal that falls after your workout):

1 large banana

PROTEIN OPTIONS:

1 cup of Egg Beaters (measured uncooked) -or-
2 scoops of whey protein (approximately 40-45 grams of protein)

Meal 2 (10:30 AM)

PROTEIN SHAKE:

Meal replacement shake such as Prolab's Naturally Lean Matrix -or-
1 scoop of protein powder such as Prolab's Protein Component mixed with 16 ounces of skim milk

GOOD FATS:

1 teaspoon of flaxseed oil

Meal 3 (12:30 PM)

CARB OPTIONS:

1 cup of brown or white rice	-or-
medium sized baked potato	-or-
medium sized sweet potato	-or-
1 cup of oatmeal (measured dry)	

VEGETABLE OPTIONS (Fibrous Carbs):

2 cup of green beans mixed with any other desired vegetable -or-
2 cup of broccoli mixed with any other desired vegetable

PROTEIN OPTIONS:

8 ounces of chicken	-or-
8 ounces of turkey	-or-
8 ounces of lean fish such as tuna, grouper, red snapper	-or-
8 ounces of 97% lean steak such as top round sirloin	

Meal 4 (3:30 PM)

PROTEIN SHAKE:

Meal replacement shake such as Prolab's Naturally Lean Matrix -or-
1 scoop of protein powder such as Prolab's Protein Component mixed with 16 ounces of skim milk

GOOD FATS:

1 teaspoon of flaxseed oil

RECOMMENDED SUPPLEMENTS:

MULTIPLE VITAMIN/
MINERAL PAKS:
PROLAB's Training Paks

MEAL REPLACEMENT
POWDERS:
PROLAB's Naturally Lean Matrix

PROTEIN POWDERS:
PROLAB's Protein Component

FLAXSEED OIL:
Spectrum's flaxseed oil as it is always kept refrigerated on the way to the retail store.

If following the Advanced Program, the following supplements may also be useful:

CREATINE:
PROLAB's Creatine Monohydrate Powder

GLUTAMINE:
PROLAB's Glutamine Powder

BEVERAGE TIPS

Many dieters can literally just blow their diets without realizing that they're doing it. The culprit? Drinking the wrong types of beverages.

Drink plenty of water daily. Your recommended fluid intake should be 0.66 x body weight in ounces per day.

Absolutely no regular sodas or fruit juices, even the ones that claim to be all natural, they contain too many simple carbs. For example, the average soda contains 40 grams of sugar while an 8-ounce serving of the average fruit juice contains between 25-35 grams of simple carbs!

Crystal Lite beverages, and decaffeinated tea/coffee are OK as long as they are used in moderation; your main beverage should be water.

Try to avoid alcohol. An occasional glass of red wine is OK provided that you are of legal drinking age.

weight. If you are gaining, cut your calories by 150 for both the lower and higher calorie diets. You'll notice that we did not cut the calories by quite as much, as your metabolism might only need a 150-calorie deficit. If you find that you are still gaining, even after the 150-calorie cut, you may decrease your calories by the additional 150 calories. Don't jump the gun! Give your body the opportunity to adjust.

EATING ON THE RUN: FAST FOODS

Today's hustle and bustle can really tax your abilities to plan and prepare. This preparation certainly includes the scheduling of food consumption. If, for one reason or another, your time constraints don't allow you to prepare all of the food you need for the day, or if you run out of food, there is a solution. You can go to a fast food restaurant. But aren't fast foods bad if you are trying to get in shape? The answer is no—as long as you choose wisely.

The rules for eating in fast food restaurants (or any other type of restaurant) are set below:

- If it is not your cheat day (see the Sunday Reward) refrain from fatty choices such as french fries.
- Drink between 8-16 ounces of water before you get to the restaurant and then drink an additional 8-16 ounces while you eat. This will prevent you from feeling hungry and falling to temptation. If you find that temptation is strong remember two things: (1) There is nothing better than being in shape. (2) You control everything that goes into your mouth. Food does not and should not control you!
- Always combine a serving of low-fat protein (in the case of fast food restaurants, this is either skinless chicken or turkey) with a small serving of carbs. Remember that if you are eating a chicken or turkey sandwich, the bread will count as the carbs.
- Salads in addition to a serving of protein and a serving of starchy carbs are always good since they provide fiber and fill you up. However, avoid using high fat/high sugar dressings.
- Refrain from using high carbohydrate sauces or mayonnaise.

Now that we know the rules of fast food eating, see the box below for some healthy meals you can choose at some of the major fast food chains.

Well, there you have it. If you find yourself in another restaurant we haven't discussed, don't panic! Just ask for a chicken plate and if it comes with skin, just take it off. Basically, if you stick to the five rules discussed above, no matter where you find yourself, you won't have a problem finding something to eat. Bon Appetit!

THE SUNDAY REWARD

For one meal each Sunday we want you to cheat on your diet. You can go to a restaurant, have a nice appetizer, a main meal and a dessert. Much more cheating than this (having two appetizers and three desserts, for instance) and you risk going backwards. You can only reward yourself in this way if you have stayed on track the rest of the week. One cheat meal a week is actually beneficial since it confuses

FAST FOOD CHOICES

In **Arby's** you can have either a Light Chicken Deluxe Sandwich with extra lettuce and tomato (no mayo) or a Light Turkey Deluxe Sandwich. They also have an excellent roast chicken salad that will not harm you unless you fill it up with high fat dressing.

In **Bennigan's** try the chicken platter, which includes a serving of spicy rice along with vegetables and two chicken breasts.

In **Boston Market** for protein you can have a serving of turkey breast or chicken breast. For carbs, you can have a small serving of steamed vegetables along with potatoes, or corn, or rice pilaf or fruit salad. If you'd rather have something quicker, then go for the chicken or turkey sandwich.

In the **Golden Corral** try the chicken (remove the skin) with their steamed rice and green beans.

In **Hardee's** order either a chicken fillet sandwich or grilled chicken salad.

In **Kentucky Fried Chicken** have a quarter chicken (no skin) for protein and a small serving of mashed potatoes, or garden rice, or red beans for carbs.

In **Long John Silver's** you may have a flavor-baked chicken or fish for protein and a small serving of plain baked potato or green beans.

In **McDonald's** you can have either a McGrilled Chicken Classic or a Chunky Chicken Salad.

In **Subway** order a Roast Turkey Breast Sub, a Veggie Sub or a Roast Beef Sub. Remember the rules that we already discussed: no extra oils or mayo etc. Also, there is no need to order a sub larger than 6 inches.

In **Taco Bell** order any of the following: a Light Chicken Burrito, or a Light Chicken Taco, or a Light Bean Burrito, or a Light Soft Taco Supreme, or a Light Taco Supreme, or a Light Taco, or a Light Soft Taco.

Finally, in **Wendy's** have either a grilled chicken sandwich or a grilled chicken salad.

your body and increases your metabolism. By cheating, you prevent your body from adjusting to the diet, which can lower your metabolism. It also removes the psychological fear that you will never be able to eat bad foods again. Having said that, we must caution that some people (us included) find it hard to go back to good dieting if they incorporate cheat foods in their diets once a week. They fall into a non-stop binging with these foods that may last for weeks. Do not feel bad if you fall into this category. Like we said, we are in this boat as well. It is natural to crave foods that are bad, considering that they taste so darn good. If you fall into this category and feel tempted or need to still build your willpower, stick to a healthy diet and stay away from cheat meals until you have reached a confident level of empowerment.

THE IMPORTANCE OF PREPARING FOOD BEFOREHAND

Preparation is crucial to the success of your dietary program. If you are not prepared, you will fail! Life is too hectic to eat five or six times a day without a little bit of preparation.

One thing you can do is to prepare your food the night before and store it in individual containers that have a section for complex or simple carbs, a place for fibrous carbs, and a place for protein. You also can prepare protein shakes the night before and store them individually in containers purchasable at the grocery store. When the following day

comes, all you have to do is take out the container that has breakfast, heat it up, and eat. Then grab the container for lunch and two protein shakes, put them in the cooler and go to work. Take a water bottle everywhere you go so you do not dehydrate while at work. When you come home, take out the container for dinner, re-heat it, eat it, and prepare the food for the following day.

COOKING TIPS

Follow the guidelines below to ensure proper food preparation:

- Eat vegetables raw or slightly steamed. If boiling be careful not to overcook or you will lose the nutritional value of the vegetables.

- Do not fry. Always broil, grill, steam or bake (broiling, grilling and steaming are better as they allow fat to drain while cooking).

- Trim all fat from meat and remove skin from poultry prior to cooking.

- Do not use salts, butter, oils, or sugar while cooking. Experiment with herbs, non-salt seasonings, lemon juice, vinegar, garlic and pepper, even a touch (1 tbsp; not a bottle) of some white or red wine. Occasional use of salsa, low sodium soy sauce, catsup, and mustard to enhance meats and vegetables is OK if used sparingly (1 tbsp). Minced white or green onions are also excellent for seasoning.

If you think you will be able to stick to the plan without being prepared, you place yourself at risk. You will either end up eating the wrong kinds of food, or missing meals. You will definitely spend more money, because eating out is not cheap. Therefore, remember to be prepared!

MEAL FREQUENCY AND WORK

Choose from among these alternatives to make sure you get your five or six meals in each day:

Have breakfast, lunch, and dinner as real meals and keep the rest of the meals as meal replacement protein shakes. Protein bars are discouraged as recent research indicates that even the low carb bars increase insulin levels by as much as a sugar loaded bar.

Have all of your meals as real meals by convincing your boss to have three 20 minute breaks instead of a full hour lunch so you can eat all of your meals.

In my experience, the more real food you eat the better the results. High-level bodybuilders know this and that is the reason that the last few weeks before a contest they will eat as much as eight real meals per day!

PROTEIN SHAKES

It's better to eat as much real food as possible, but if you are too busy to fix four to six real meals, you can substitute meals with a shake. You can have either a meal replacement packet mixed with water or a scoop of protein mixed in skim milk with a teaspoon

of flaxseed oil (refer to the supplements section for more information). However, make sure that you eat at least two real meals a day (three being preferred).

EMOTIONAL EATING

In our fast-paced, high-stress society, many people resort to emotional eating for comfort. This is a dangerous activity; if this happens very often, the weight will begin to pile on. Also dangerous is the fact that emotional eating usually occurs at night after work.

If you feel like you engage in emotional eating, remember the reasons why you embarked in this program on the first place. Also, keep in mind that overeating is not going to solve any problems and will prevent you from getting the results you deserve. Always ask yourself: "Am I eating this because my body needs it or because I need it emotionally?" Stop to think about what is most important for you. Is it the food or your goals? If it's late at night, go to bed and rest assured that the craving will go away by the time the morning comes.

NOTES ON SUPPLEMENTATION

- A good multiple vitamin and mineral formula taken preferably with your post-workout meal or at breakfast on non-workout days to avoid any nutritional deficiencies. Make sure that it has at least 500mg of calcium, or get a separate calcium supplement such as calcium citrate, which is best absorbed by the body.

- Chromium Picolinate (200 mcg) also with the post-workout meal or at breakfast. This mineral is good for increasing acceptance of insulin. A good insulin sensitivity is necessary in order to optimize the fat burning process. Note: Some multiple vitamin/mineral formulas already have this, so check the label.

- 1000 mg of Vitamin C three times a day. Start with only 500mg and increase the dosage by 500mg per week until you reach the 3000mg total. This is in order to avoid any stomach problems. Vitamin C is fantastic at reducing cortisol levels, which is the stress hormone released by the adrenal glands that eats muscle and stores fat.

- Whey Protein Shakes or Meal Replacement Shakes like Prolab's Naturally Lean Matrix, which is based on complex carbohydrates and a blend of different proteins consisting of a 40/40/20 macronutrient ratio. It contains 20 grams of carbs, 20 grams of proteins and 4 grams of good fats making it the perfect meal replacement supplement for this program. The product is also instantized: it requires no blender just some water and a spoon and the taste is fantastic.

Part II

The Exercises

Here are all the exercises you will need to sculpt the body of your dreams. We've given you stretches to warm up and cool down, challenging exercises for every body part, combination exercises for the most efficient workouts, and alternative exercises you can do on stack machines if you prefer.

Chapter 3

Warm Up and Stretch Out

The pre-workout warm up and post-workout stretch are vital components of your Body Sculpting Bible *EXPRESS* Workout. And they don't require a lot of time—just a few minutes. The next few pages will show you how to warm up most effectively for your workout and how to stretch out your muscles to prevent injury.

THE BODY SCULPTING BIBLE EXPRESS

WARM UP BEFORE YOU WORKOUT

Research indicates that you should perform an active warm up before you begin a workout. The purposes of the warm up are many: to increase blood flow to the muscles you will be working; to increase your heart-rate; to increase your body temperature and therefore warm your joints and improve your flexibility; and to prepare

3

your neuromuscular system for the movements you will need to perform.

The best way to warm up for the Body Sculpting *EXPRESS* Workout is to perform about five minutes of a combination of squats, jumping jacks, and jogging or fast walking. In your warm up try to use all of the muscles you will be working during your *EXPRESS* workout, including your arms.

WHEN TO STRETCH

While there's scant evidence that static stretching (the type of stretch that involves holding a stretched position for a number of seconds with no bouncing) before your workout prevents injury, you can do a few pre-workout stretches that are dynamic. Dynamic stretches involve performing several repetitions of bringing a muscle quickly into a stretched position and then immediately releasing it. This type of stretching helps to prepare your muscles for the workout ahead.

Recent research strongly indicates that the best and safest time to do static stretching is at the end of the workout. This is when your muscles are warm due to increased blood flow; therefore it is the best time to elongate them. In addition there's less risk of causing injury by overstretching when the muscles are warm. In contrast, if you perform static stretches on cold muscles (for example first thing in the morning), your range of motion is much more limited and you risk pushing the stretch too far and injuring the muscle or connective tissues.

HOW TO PERFORM THE STATIC STRETCH

Begin your static stretch by inhaling from your diaphragm (the base of your lungs) rather than from your chest (a helpful mental image is to imagine you are inflating a balloon with your breathing). As you move into the stretch position, exhale. Go deep enough into a stretch to feel tension in the muscles you are stretching. Never force a stretch. Hold the stretch position for 10 to 30 seconds before releasing. Continue to breathe deeply while in the stretch position. As you hold the stretch, you will begin to feel your muscles moving from a state of tension to relaxation. At this point, you can try to take the stretch a bit deeper. It is normal to feel some discomfort during the initial moments of the stress; if you feel any pain however, ease up on the stretch immediately.

YOUR STRETCH PROGRAM

The stretches that appear on the following pages can be done dynamically before your workout, or statically afterwards. Before your workout, perform several repetitions of each stretch, holding each one for only 1 to 3 seconds. After your workout, perform one repetition of each stretch but hold without bouncing for as long as 30 seconds.

LOWER BACK STRETCH

This stretch is a yoga favorite, also known as the cat stretch. It warms up and stretches the lower back and abdominal muscles.

TECHNIQUE AND FORM

1 Begin on your hands and knees with your back slightly curved.

2 Exhale as you round your back and pull your abdominals up into your spine.

TRAINER'S TIPS

Make sure your wrists are under your shoulders and your knees are directly under your hips.

UPPER BACK AND BICEPS STRETCH

This terrific stretch is for the muscles in the mid- and upper-back and the front of your arms.

TECHNIQUE AND FORM

1 Start in a standing position.

2 Interlock your fingers and exhale as you press your arms forward (palms facing front). Pull your abs into your spine and round your chest.

TRAINER'S TIPS

✪ Keep your knees slightly bent as you perform the stretch.

✪ Your legs should remain still while you stretch. Only your arms and torso move.

CHEST STRETCH

This stretch opens the muscles in your chest, improving your posture and preventing injury.

TECHNIQUE AND FORM

1 Stand facing a wall, with your right arm extended and hand pressed against the wall.

2 Lean into the wall and then twist your torso away from it, until you feel the stretch in the right side of your chest and upper arm.

TRAINER'S TIPS

⊗ If your shoulder hurts, release the stretch immediately.

STANDING HAMSTRING STRETCH

This stretch relieves tension in the hamstring muscles at the back of your legs. These muscles tend to be tight in most people, so be sure to ease into the stretch position slowly.

TECHNIQUE AND FORM

1 Begin in the standing position. Bend from the waist, pulling your abs in to your spine. At the same time extend your left leg, while you bend your right knee. (Your weight should rest on the heel of your left foot.)

2 Place your hands on your left thigh and press into the stretch position.

3 Repeat on your other leg.

TRAINER'S TIPS

Try not to lock out your leg as you stretch—always maintain a slight bend in the knee.

You can make this stretch more intense by varying the position of the leg being stretched. Try placing it up on a bench or a chair as you stretch.

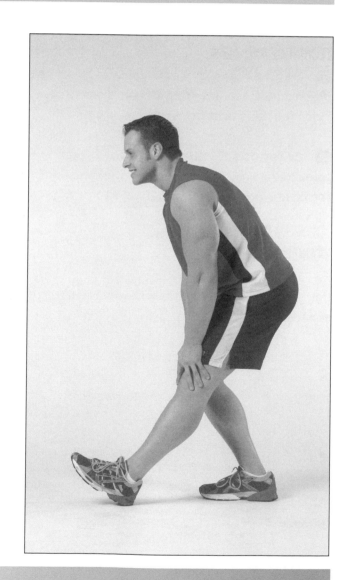

SEATED INNER THIGH STRETCH

Many people have limited flexibility in their inner thighs, so take care not to overstretch.

TECHNIQUE AND FORM

1 Sit on the floor or mat with your heels pressed together and your knees out to the side. Place your hands around your ankles.

2 As you exhale, press your elbows against your thighs, trying to press your thighs closer to the floor.

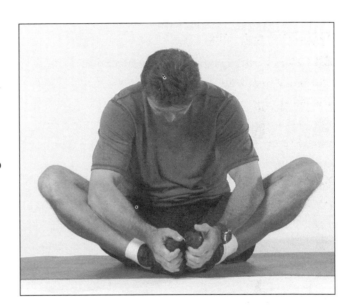

TRAINER'S TIPS

⊗ Really think about pressing your thighs down against the floor as you execute the stretch.

⊗ This is a great stretch to have an assistant. Your helper kneels behind you and gently but firmly presses his hands against your thighs, lowering them toward the floor.

THIGH STRETCH

The classic quadriceps stretch for the front of your thighs can change in intensity depending upon the angle of the stretch.

TECHNIQUE AND FORM

1   Stand, supporting yourself against a wall or by holding onto a pole.

2   Bend your opposite leg behind you, bringing your heel toward your buttocks.

3   Grasp your ankle with your free hand and press in until you feel the stretch in the front of your thigh. Repeat with your other leg.

TRAINER'S TIPS

✪   Keep your abdominals engaged throughout this stretch.

✪   To intensify the stretch you can lean slightly forward from the hips.

✪   Make sure your knee is in line with your hips and not out to the side.

✪   As an extra balance challenge, try this exercise without a support. If you focus your eyes on a point straight ahead of you, you will increase your ability to balance.

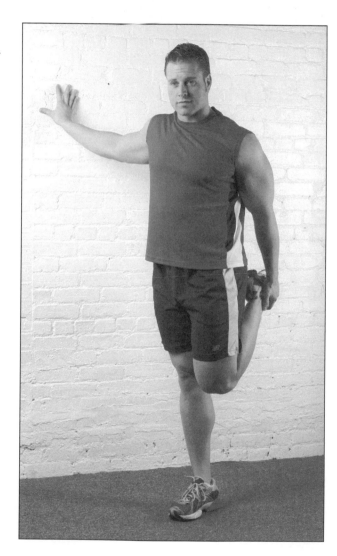

STANDING CALF STRETCH

This stretches the lower muscles in the back of your leg that can cramp up and make you prone to injury if too tight.

TECHNIQUE AND FORM

1 Stand straight with your left knee bent about one foot in front of you and your right leg extended a little more than one foot behind your body.

2 Place your hands on your left thigh as you lean slightly forward from the hips and press your right heel into the floor.

3 Repeat with your other leg.

TRAINER'S TIPS

Breathe deeply into the stretch. Make sure that your heel is in contact with the floor. If you can't touch the back heel down, bring your back leg in closer to your body.

Keep your head in line with your neck and look straight ahead. Your shoulders should be pulled back and pressed down as you perform this stretch.

TRICEPS STRETCH

When you perform the triceps stretch for the back of your arms, make sure that you concentrate on reaching your hand down your back as you press your elbow in.

TECHNIQUE AND FORM

1 Stand or sit cross-legged.

2 Reach your right arm straight overhead, then bend it so that your right hand is reaching down your back.

3 Use your left hand to press your right elbow close to your head; at the same time reach down your back with your right hand.

4 Repeat with your other arm.

TRAINER'S TIPS

⊗ Exhale deeply as you reach your hand down your back.

⊗ Make sure your fingers remain unclenched.

SHOULDER STRETCH

This is an excellent way to stretch the shoulders and thus prevent injury.

TECHNIQUE AND FORM

1 Stand straight. Grasp one of your elbows with the opposite hand.

2 Without moving your torso, pull your arm as far as possible toward your body.

3 Repeat with your other arm.

TRAINER'S TIPS

✪ Keep your arm parallel to the floor as you pull it toward your body.

✪ Keep your legs about shoulder width apart for balance and support.

Chapter 4
Back and Chest

This chapter includes exercises for two of your body's large muscle groups—the back and chest. Your back and chest actually contain several muscles and are ideal to train in a time-efficient workout like the *EXPRESS* workout. When you exercise your back, you train not only the specific back muscles such as the rhomboids, traps, and lats, but you also train the smaller assisting muscles in your arms—the biceps and deltoids. Likewise, when you train your chest, in addition to working the pectoralis major and minor (the chest muscles) you build the helping muscles in the arms: the triceps and the anterior delts. Most men tend to focus on strengthening their chest muscles, and neglect their back muscles. It's important to work both of these opposing muscle groups for balance, injury prevention, optimum strength, and appearance. A strong, muscular back helps your waist look smaller and makes you look more muscular that you really are.

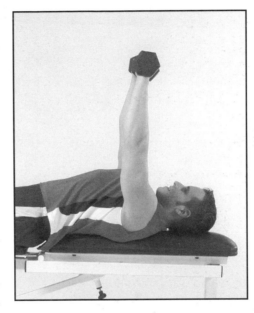

THE BODY SCULPTING BIBLE
EXPRESS

4

ONE-ARM ROW—PALMS FACING TORSO

The one-arm row is a variation of the two-arm bent-over row. It involves less lower-back involvement and is particularly suited for people with back problems, or who do not yet have strong enough abdominal and other core muscles to lift two weights in good form. For a similar machine exercise, try the Two-Arm Row or the Wide Grip Pulldowns.

TECHNIQUE AND FORM

1 Place your right knee and right hand on a bench or chair for support.

2 Bend at the waist until your upper body is close to parallel to the bench.

3 Lean into your right hand to help support your body weight. You will be training the left side of your back.

4 Pick up a weight with your left hand so that your palm faces your torso. Continue to support your back with your right side. This will be your starting position.

5 Lift your left elbow up toward the ceiling as you exhale. Squeeze and hold in the top position for a second.

6 Slowly lower back to the starting position as you inhale.

7 Repeat for desired number of repetitions.

8 Switch sides and perform the same exercise for the right side of your back.

TRAINER'S TIPS

Be sure to keep your abdominals pulled in tight as you lift the weight.

Keep your arm right next to your side, your head in line with your spine, and look straight ahead throughout the exercise.

Avoid twisting or turning your torso.

ONE-ARM ROW—PALMS FACING TORSO

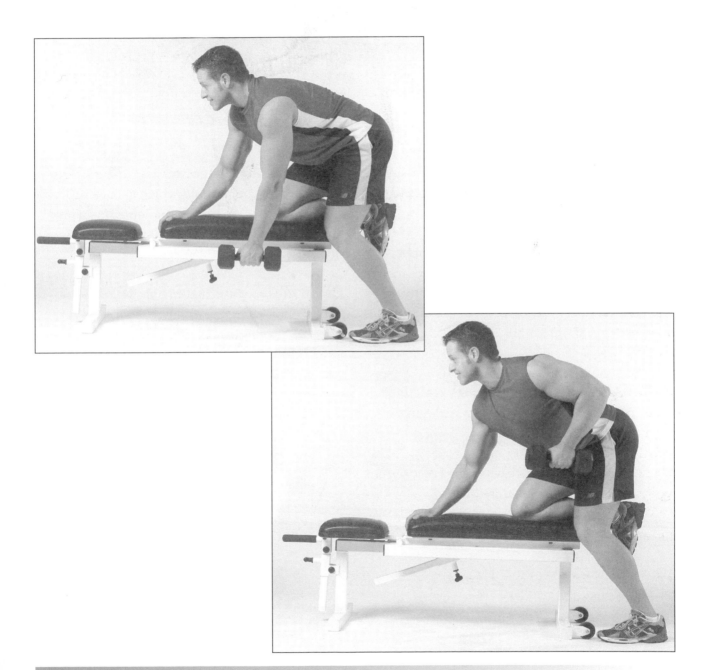

INCLINE DUMBBELL BENCH PRESS

The incline dumbbell press targets your upper chest muscles. Performing this exercise with dumbbells requires your stabilizer muscles to keep the weights balanced. A machine alternate for this exercise is the Bench Press Machine.

TECHNIQUE AND FORM

1 With dumbbells on your thighs, thrust one leg up, leveraging one dumbbell up to your chest.

2 Immediately thrust the second dumbbell upward at the same time as you allow momentum and the dumbbells to guide you back into an inclined position. Use your abdominal muscles to ease you into position.

3 Press the weights straight up to the ceiling. Keep your chest lifted, your elbows out and wide, and your forearms perpendicular to the floor.

4 Lower the weights slowly, making sure your body remains in good alignment.

TRAINER'S TIPS

As you perform the exercise, make sure that you pull your shoulder blades back against the bench (this is called retraction). This allows your chest to do more work than your shoulders.

At the top of the movement you have the option of touching the dumbbells together and squeezing your chest or of pressing the weights straight up. As a variation, you can also turn your palms toward each other at the top of the movement.

INCLINE DUMBBELL BENCH PRESS

ONE-ARM ROW—PALMS FACING REAR

The one-arm row is a variation of the two-arm bent-over row. It involves less lower-back involvement and is particularly suited for people with back problems, or who do not yet have strong enough abdominal and other core muscles to lift two weights in good form. For a similar machine ezxercise, try the Two-Arm Row Machine or the Wide Grip Pulldowns.

TECHNIQUE AND FORM

1 Place your right knee and right hand on a bench or chair for support.

2 Bend at the waist until your upper body is close to parallel to the bench.

3 Lean into your right hand to help support your bodyweight. You will be training the left side of your back.

4 Pick up a weight with your left hand so that your palm faces to the rear. Continue to support your back with your right side. This will be your starting position.

5 Lift your left elbow up toward the ceiling as you exhale. Squeeze and hold in the top position for a second.

6 Slowly lower back to the starting position as you inhale.

7 Repeat for desired number of repetitions.

8 Switch sides and perform the same exercise for the right side of your back.

TRAINER'S TIPS

Be sure to keep your abdominals pulled in tight as you lift the weight.

Keep your arm right next to your side, your head in line with your spine, and look straight ahead throughout the exercise.

Avoid twisting or turning your torso.

ONE-ARM ROW—PALMS FACING REAR

FLAT DUMBBELL BENCH PRESS

This exercise focuses on the muscles in the middle of your chest. A machine alternate for this exercise is the Bench Press Machine.

TECHNIQUE AND FORM

1 With dumbbells on your thighs, thrust one leg up, leveraging one dumbbell up to your chest.

2 Immediately thrust the second dumbbell upward at the same time as you allow momentum and the dumbbells to guide you back into a lying position. Use your abdominal muscles to ease you into position.

3 Keep your back flat by pulling your abdominals in.

4 Beginning from this position, where your elbows are slightly lower than the bench, press the weights straight up toward the ceiling, keeping your chest lifted, your elbows out and wide, and your forearms perpendicular to the floor.

5 Lower the weights slowly, making sure you keep your back pressed into the bench.

TRAINER'S TIPS

✪ As you perform the exercise, make sure that you pull your shoulder blades back against the bench (this is called retraction). This allows your chest to do more work than your shoulders.

✪ At the top of the movement you have the option of touching the dumbbells together and squeezing your chest or of pressing them straight up. As a variation, you can also turn your palms toward each other at the top of the movement.

✪ Variety is the spice of exercise, so try the exercise different ways to keep your muscles alert and challenged.

✪ Always keep your forearms perpendicular to the floor.

FLAT DUMBBELL BENCH PRESS

Chapter 5

Arms

The exercises in this chapter work your biceps and triceps. Pay particular attention to your form in all of these exercises—the slightest variations in position can have great impact on the results you'll experience. Therefore, if big arms are your goal, form should be your top priority.

THE BODY SCULPTING BIBLE EXPRESS

5

DUMBBELL CURLS

These exercises are for the biceps; you can also perform them with a barbell instead of dumbbells if you want to go heavy on the weights but protect your wrists. There are two machine alternates for this exercise: the Biceps Curl Machine and the High Pulley Cable Curl Machine.

TECHNIQUE AND FORM

1 Stand in a neutral position with your abs held in and a natural curve to your spine. Hold a dumbbell in each hand. Your arms are slightly bent at the elbows and your palms face forward.

2 Slowly curl the dumbbells up toward your shoulders, without moving your elbows.

3 Once you reach the top position, hold for a moment contracting your biceps as hard as you can, before returning to the starting position.

TRAINER'S TIPS

Be careful not to sway back or forward while executing the curl. If you do, you may be using weight that is too heavy.

Make sure your arms are not locked out when in the down position. This will place too much pressure on your biceps and make you vulnerable to injury.

Perform the biceps curls carefully, not using momentum to lift the weights.

DUMBBELL CURLS

LYING DUMBBELL TRICEPS EXTENSION

The triceps are three muscles located at the back of your upper arm. This exercise focuses on the outer muscles. You can also perform it in a standing position, but lying down is the safest alternative. There are two machines that provide similar muscle stimulation: the Triceps Extension Machine and the Triceps Pushdown Machine.

TECHNIQUE AND FORM

1 Lie down on your back, and with a dumbbell in each hand, press your arms toward the ceiling. Your palms should face each other.

2 Bend your elbows to lower the dumbbells toward your head. The upper part of your arms should remain frozen in place. Only your forearms move during this exercise.

3 Once the weights come close to your forehead, slowly press them back up to the starting position with your arms extended.

4 Hold this position and contract your triceps hard.

TRAINER'S TIPS

✪ Concentrate on your form and on accentuating the contraction when you extend your arms; this will more completely stimulate your muscles.

✪ Even though you are straightening your arms over your head, always maintain a slight bend to your elbows for safety.

✪ You can maintain more tension in your triceps by keeping your upper arms slanted on an angle with your head.

LYING DUMBBELL TRICEPS EXTENSION

HAMMER CURLS

The hammer curl works the outer biceps and forearms. It is similar to the dumbbell curl, except it is performed with your palms facing each other.

TECHNIQUE AND FORM

1 Stand in a neutral alignment (your body straight, head in line with your spine, knees slightly bent and shoulder-width apart, and a natural curve to your lower back). Hold a weight in each hand with your palms facing each other.

2 Exhale and curl the dumbbells up toward your shoulders. Make sure you keep your elbows at your sides and pointed at the ground throughout the exercise.

3 At the top position, contract your biceps and forearm muscles as hard as you can and hold for a couple of seconds.

TRAINER'S TIPS

To keep your body straight, pull in your abdominal muscles, stick out your chest, and keep your shoulders squared.

You can perform this exercise while seated to make it more of an isolation exercise. This position will be more challenging for the biceps muscles.

HAMMER CURLS

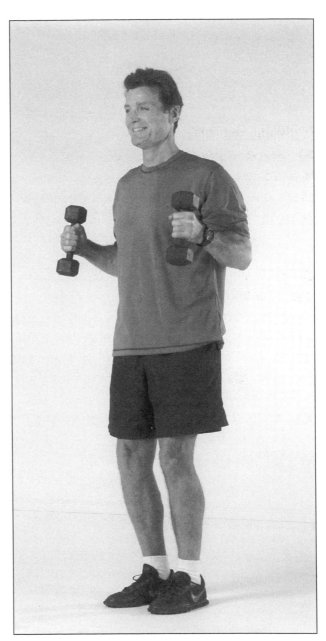

OVERHEAD DUMBBELL TRICEPS EXTENSION

This exercise targets the middle and inner triceps muscles. It can be performed either seated or standing.

TECHNIQUE AND FORM

1 Begin in a seated or standing position. If seated, make sure that your back is flat against the backpad at all times. If standing, make sure that your abs are pulled in, your knees are slightly bent, and your legs are shoulder width apart for balance and support.

2 Hold the dumbbell with both hands over your head, grasping it so that you get an even grip with both hands. (This is important; if your grip is uneven, you will be working out one arm more than the other.)

3 Lower the dumbbell while keeping your elbows pointed to the ceiling.

4 Exhale as you press the dumbbell back up to the top position.

5 At the top position, contract the triceps as hard as you can and hold for a couple of seconds before lowering.

TRAINER'S TIPS

⊗ Throughout the exercise make sure your elbows are in close to your head and pointed up at the ceiling. This ensures full range of motion for the triceps.

⊗ When you extend your arms, maintain a slight bend to the elbows to avoid locking out at the joint.

⊗ Keep your head in line with your spine. Throughout the exercise avoid looking down.

OVERHEAD DUMBBELL TRICEPS EXTENSION

Chapter 6
Shoulders and Calves

In this chapter we will cover the exercises that target your shoulders and calf muscles. All of these muscle groups must be trained correctly in order to have a cut and symmetrical upper and lower body. Big shoulders help make you look wider and give your body a nice three-dimensional look. Large calves make your upper thighs look bigger and your legs look powerful.

Since the shoulder muscles are smaller and weaker, you may have to use lighter weights when working with them. Again, concentrate on good form. In contrast, the calves are usually strong and can handle heavy weights.

THE BODY SCULPTING BIBLE EXPRESS

6

ONE-LEGGED DUMBBELL CALF RAISES

This exercise can be performed on the floor, but for optimal range of motion, perform it off of a step, bench, or calf block. A machine alternate to this exercise is the Calf Raise Machine.

TECHNIQUE AND FORM

1 Grasp a dumbbell with your left hand and position the balls of your right foot on a calf block or a raised platform with the heels extending off. The toes should be facing forward.

2 Place your right hand on a fixed object such as a beam on a squat rack in order to keep your body balanced. Lift your left leg by bending at the knee.

3 Raise the heels of your right leg by extending the ankles as high as possible as you contract the calves. Exhale as you perform this movement and contract at the top for a second.

4 Lower the heels by bending the ankles until the calves are fully stretched. Inhale as you perform this portion of the movement.

5 Repeat for the recommended amount of repetitions. When you are done with the right leg, perform the exercise with the left leg.

TRAINER'S TIPS

For help balancing, place your right hand on a fixed object such as a beam on a squat rack.

Instead of a bench, you may use the dumbbells themselves to perform this exercise.

ONE-LEGGED DUMBBELL CALF RAISES

DUMBBELL SHOULDER PRESS

The dumbbell shoulder press works the front and laterals of the shoulders. It's a great exercise that not only challenges the shoulders, but works on your balance and stability too.

TECHNIQUE AND FORM

1 Stand in neutral position, with your knees slightly bent and your feet shoulder width apart for support. Hold a dumbbell in each hand over your shoulders. Your palms should face forward and your elbows should be at a 90 degree angle.

2 Exhale as you press the dumbbells straight up in a controlled smooth motion.

3 Once you reach the top (your arms should remain slightly bent at the elbows), hold for a moment before lowering slowly down back to a 90 degree angle.

TRAINER'S TIPS

✪ Throughout the exercise make sure you keep your arms wide, your head in line with your spine, and your back straight.

✪ If you find you are swaying either forward or backward, you need to adjust your form or go lighter weights.

✪ Concentrate on keeping your elbows as wide as possible throughout the exercise.

✪ It is unnecessary to touch the weights together at the top of the movement. This may actually injure your rotator cuff muscles.

DUMBBELL SHOULDER PRESS

TWO-LEGGED DUMBBELL CALF RAISES

This exercise can be performed on the floor, but for optimal range of motion perform it off of a step, bench, or calf block. It can be performed either one leg at a time or with both legs simultaneously. A machine alternate to this exercise is the Calf Raise Machine.

TECHNIQUE AND FORM -

1 Stand with your torso upright holding two dumbbells in your hands by your sides. This will be your starting position.

2 With the toes pointing either straight, inwards, or outwards, raise the heels off the floor as you exhale by contracting the calves. Hold the top contraction for a second.

3 As you inhale, go back to the starting position by slowly lowering the heels.

TRAINER'S TIPS

For this exercise you won't be able to achieve a full stretch at the bottom without a platform. The exercise is effective nonetheless. As you become stronger, you may need to use wrist wraps to avoid having dumbbells slip from your hands.

Instead of a bench, you may use the dumbbells themselves to perform this exercise.

TWO-LEGGED DUMBBELL CALF RAISES

VARIATION

BENT-OVER LATERAL RAISES

This is an awesome exercise that targets the back of the shoulders (the rear delts), thus providing a full, muscular, three-dimensional appearance to the shoulders. A machine alternate to this exercise is the Reverse Fly Machine.

TECHNIQUE AND FORM

1 Stand in neutral position, then bend over at your hips. Bend your knees, and keep your back straight and parallel to the floor.

2 Lift the dumbbells out to the sides of your body to shoulder height—keeping your arms slightly bent at the elbows.

3 When you reach the top position, hold for a moment before returning to the start position.

TRAINER'S TIPS

To help keep your back straight throughout the exercise pull your abdominals in tight.

BENT-OVER
LATERAL RAISES

Chapter 7
Lower Body and Abs

Men often neglect the muscles of the legs, instead focusing on their upper bodies. It is important to perform workouts for both your upper and lower body for overall balance, aesthetics, and strength. Did you know that working the muscles in your legs also stimulates testosterone release, which helps improve your overall muscle tone?

The core, primarily your abdominals and lower back muscles, drives all of your movement and powers your legs and arms. It is the part of your body that stabilizes, holding you in balance. It is your body's powerhouse and deserves special attention. Many of us have unbalanced cores from over-doing abdominal exercises and neglecting exercises that also strengthen the lower back. Imbalances can lead to back pain and injury. The Lying Leg Raises featured here for your off days work both the abs and the lower back muscles, and the Crunches primarily work the fronts of your abs.

THE BODY SCULPTING BIBLE EXPRESS

7

DUMBBELL SQUATS

The squat is one of the most effective and efficient exercises you can do for many of the muscles in the legs, including your glutes, hamstrings, and quadriceps. Not only do squats help define legs, they involve recruitment of your core muscles and work balance and stability as well. A machine alternate to this exercise is the Leg Extension Machine.

TECHNIQUE AND FORM

1 Stand in a neutral position, with your feet about hips width apart. Hold a dumbbell in each hand.

2 Bend at your knees and press your hips out behind you.

3 Lower into the squat position (coming no lower than the point where your thighs are parallel to the floor any lower and your risk knee injury).

4 Exhale, pull your abdominals in and slowly come up to the standing position.

5 Inhale and lower back down to the squat position.

TRAINER'S TIPS

✪ Keep your body weight centered over your heels rather than your toes. This will help you to be in the right position when you squat down.

✪ Keep your knees in line with your toes.

DUMBBELL SQUATS

STATIC DUMBBELL LUNGES

The lunge also works all the major muscles of your lower body, and is more challenging than the squat for balance. A machine alternate to this exercise is the Leg Extention Machine.

TECHNIQUE AND FORM

1 Stand in neutral position with your legs about shoulder width apart.

2 Step forward with you right leg. Keep your head, shoulders, and hips in alignment.

3 Bend both legs so that your right knee makes a 90 degree angle with the floor, and your left knee comes close to the floor.

4 Lift up and return to the starting position. As you lift make sure you push off with the right foot.

5 Repeat the desired number of repetitions on the right leg before switching to the left leg.

TRAINER'S TIPS

✪ Concentrate on keeping your back straight throughout the lunge; avoid leaning forward.

✪ Make sure you bend your back leg so that it almost touches the floor it is far better to perform this exercise slowly in a full range of motion than to rush through it and come down only half-way.

STATIC
DUMBBELL LUNGES

WIDE-STANCE DUMBBELL SQUATS

The wide-stance squat is similar to the dumbbell squat, but your legs are wider apart causing greater emphasis on your inner quads and inner thighs.

TECHNIQUE AND FORM

1 Stand in neutral position, with your feet one and a half times wider than your shoulders and your toes pointed to the side. Hold a dumbbell in each hand.

2 Bend at your knees and press your hips out behind you.

3 Inhale as you lower into the squat position. Go no lower than the point where your thighs are parallel to the floor. Any lower and you risk knee injury.

4 Exhale, pull your abdominals in, and slowly come up to the standing position.

5 Inhale and lower back down to the squat position.

TRAINER'S TIPS

Be careful not too take too wide of a stance, as this may injure your inner thighs or knees.

Keep your back straight and your head up in line with your spine throughout the squat.

WIDE-STANCE DUMBBELL SQUATS

DUMBBELL STIFF-LEGGED DEADLIFTS

This exercise targets both the hamstring muscles at the back of your legs and your lower back muscles. However, if you suffer from lower back injury, this exercise is not recommended because it may re-injure a weakened back by the strain it places on the back muscles. A machine alternate to this exercise is the Lying Leg Curl Machine.

TECHNIQUE AND FORM

1 Stand in neutral position with a weight in each hand, your feet shoulder width apart pointing straight ahead, and your legs locked out.

2 Bend from your waist, keeping your legs locked out and your arms hanging down in front of your thighs. Your palms should be turned toward your body.

3 Look straight ahead as you bend over. Lower until your upper body is almost parallel to the floor and the dumbbells are below your knees.

4 Slowly straighten to the starting position.

TRAINER'S TIPS

❂ It is essential that you keep your back flat as a table as you lower. Pulling your abdominals in and looking straight ahead will help you to maintain proper form.

❂ Focus on your hamstrings by thinking about the back of your legs.

❂ You can use a barbell to protect your wrists.

DUMBBELL STIFF-LEGGED DEADLIFTS

VARIATION

LYING LEG RAISES

This exercise focuses on the lower abdominals and also helps to strengthen the lower back. It must be done properly; if done incorrectly you can injure your lower back. Focus is essential.

TECHNIQUE AND FORM

1 Lie on your back with your legs straight and flat on the floor.

2 Place your hands face down under your buttocks, fingertips facing each other to support your lower back. Also, bend your knees slightly.

3 Lift your legs a few inches off the ground and hold. (Go higher if you need to avoid feeling pain in your lower back.)

4 Squeeze your abs as hard as you can and hold for a couple of seconds.

5 Slowly lower your legs closer to the floor.

TRAINER'S TIPS

Think, think, and think about this exercise as you do it. Focus and feel your abs working as you raise your legs up.

If you feel any pain in your lower back, stop.

LYING
LEG RAISES

CRUNCHES

Although there are plenty of trendy abdominal exercises around these days, the basic crunch remains one of the most effective for the abs.

TECHNIQUE AND FORM

1 Lay down on your back with your knees bent and your feet flat on the floor.

2 Cross your hands in front of your chest (beginner) or bend them behind your head (intermediate).

3 Pull your abs in and exhale as you move your chest up toward your knees.

4 At the top position, contract your abs as hard as you can and hold for a couple of seconds.

5 Return to the lower position, without letting your shoulders touch the floor, and immediately begin the next repetition.

TRAINER'S TIPS

How high you come up is not important. Focus on getting the strongest contraction in your abs.

If you place a folded bath towel under your lower back you can increase the range of motion of the crunch and therefore achieve more muscle stimulation.

CRUNCHES

VARIATION

THE
BICYCLE

This exercise, commonly known as the bicycle, is very effective when done properly. In a study conducted by the American Council on Exercise, it was found to be one of the most effective exercises you can do to stimulate the muscle fibers in the abdominal area.

TECHNIQUE AND FORM

1 Lie on your back, keeping your hands behind your head and your knees bent.

2 Crunch up as you start, twisting your right side toward your left knee and extending your right leg.

3 Switch sides immediately, bringing your right knee in as you extend your left leg.

TRAINER'S TIPS

🔄 Try to keep your back pressed against the floor; avoid having it arch up.

🔄 The extended leg should be a few inches off the floor. If you place it too close to the floor you can strain your back.

🔄 When you twist toward your knee actively think about twisting with your waist, rather than with your elbow. If you feel that you are pulling against your neck, you may be using your arms rather than your waist to twist.

THE BICYCLE

THE PLANK

A staple of yoga classes, the plank works the deep internal muscles of your core, including your back. (Maintaining the plank position is also a tough workout for your arms and shoulders.)

TECHNIQUE AND FORM

1 Lie on your stomach with your forearms against the floor and your legs extended behind you.

2 Lift your body up, keeping your forearms against the floor. Make sure that you keep your back as straight as possible. Avoid arching or curving your back.

3 Hold the position for 10 seconds.

4 Lift the right arm and left leg simultaneously and hold for five seconds.

5 Switch sides and hold for five seconds.

6 Relax into the starting position.

TRAINER'S TIPS

If your core isn't strong enough to maintain a neutral position for your spine, you may lift your hips up a bit until you get stronger.

Make sure you keep your head in line with your spine throughout this exercise.

THE
PLANK

V-KNEE

This very challenging exercise is more advanced; work up to it.

TECHNIQUE AND FORM

1   Sit with your legs straight out in front and your arms bent at the elbows. Your palms should be pressed against the floor.

2   Lean back and bring your legs up, balancing on your sit bones. Feel the contraction in your abdominals.

3   Slowly bring your knees in toward your chest at the same time as you lift your chest toward your knees.

TRAINER'S TIPS

✪   To increase the intensity of this exercise you can try performing it with your hands off the floor and out in front of you. You also can add a twist to your torso as you lift. These alternatives should only be performed when you have sufficient core strength to perform the basic exercise.

V-KNEE

SET UP

VARIATION

LOWER BACK EXTENSION

This exercise, also known as the Cobra or Sphinx, is a great strengthener of the erector spinae muscles in your lower back.

TECHNIQUE AND FORM

1 Lie on your stomach with your legs extended behind you and your hands pressed against the floor.

2 Exhale and lift your torso by straightening your arms.

3 Hold that position for a couple of seconds.

TRAINER'S TIPS

Keep your hips in contact with the floor throughout the exercise.

If you feel any pain in your back, do not continue this exercise.

If you cannot extend your arms fully, you can keep your forearms on the floor and lift your chest.

LOWER
BACK EXTENSION

Chapter 8

Combination Exercises

Get ready for some of the most challenging, heart-pumping exercises you've ever done! While traditional toning exercises focus primarily on one or two muscle groups (for example, the dumbbell row for your mid-back), the combo exercises featured in this chapter work several muscles simultaneously. In most, you will be strengthening your legs and your upper body at the same time. The result? An exercise that efficiently sculpts your upper and lower body simultaneously. And there are additional benefits: because these exercises are all free-weight based, you will be improving balance and strengthening your all-important core muscles as well. As you'll see, the combo exercises are especially suited for an overall body workout that is short on time, but long on intensity.

Because these exercises involve a lot more movement and work more muscles than traditional weight-lifting with machines, you will probably have to use dumbbells that are a bit lighter than you normally would—especially when you first start out. If you find that you are having trouble balancing or performing the exercises in good form, go lighter.

THE BODY SCULPTING BIBLE

EXPRESS

8

SQUATS WITH DUMBBELL ROWS

This exercise pairs the squat for your hamstrings, quadriceps, and gluteals with the row for your back.

TECHNIQUE AND FORM

1 Begin in a standing position with your body in neutral form, your feet approximately shoulder width apart. Hold a dumbbell in each hand and hold your arms down by your sides.

2 Inhale and lower into the squat position with your knees bent, your hips pressed out behind you, and your thighs no lower than parallel to the floor. As you lower, your arms slowly extend in front of your legs at an angle.

3 Exhale and pull your abdominals in toward your spine as you straighten your legs. At the same time as you straighten, bend your arms to bring the weights in toward your waist, pulling your elbows behind you.

4 Extend your arms and lower your body back down into the starting position.

TRAINER'S TIPS

As you begin to lift, make sure that your body weight is balanced over the heels of your feet rather than the toes. A good way to check this is to lift your toes while you are in the squat-ready position to see if you remain balanced. If you can't balance, try shifting your weight back toward your heels.

Your knees should be in line with your toes (it doesn't matter whether your legs are slightly turned out or straight ahead).

Keep your head in line with your spine look straight ahead as you lift and perform the row.

SQUATS WITH DUMBBELL ROWS

LUNGES WITH OVERHEAD PRESS

You'll feel your heart rate climb with the lunge/overhead press combo, so go easy on the weights, especially if this type of exercise is new to you.

TECHNIQUE AND FORM

1 Stand straight, with a natural curve to your back and a dumbbell in each hand at shoulder height.

2 Step forward with your right leg, bending your right knee until it is perpendicular to the floor. At the same time, bend your left knee so that it comes close to the floor.

3 As you step forward with your right leg, press the weights up and over your head.

4 Straighten to the starting position, bringing your right leg back to meet your left leg, as you also lower the weights to your shoulders.

5 Perform same exercise beginning with the left leg.

TRAINER'S TIPS

⊗ Keep your abdominals pulled in tight for this exercise. It will help you remain balanced.

⊗ If you feel any sharp pain in your shoulders, switch to lighter weights.

⊗ Keep your head straight.

LUNGES WITH OVERHEAD PRESS

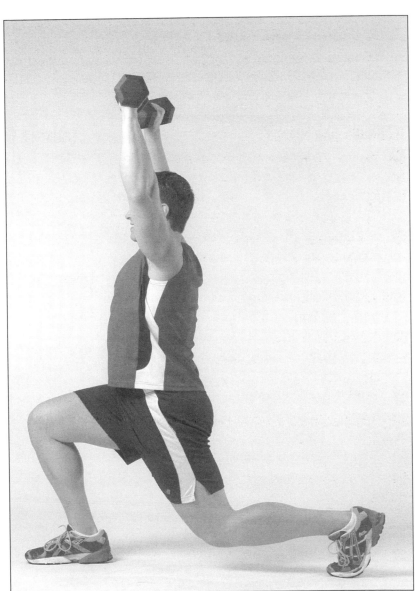

WIDE SQUATS WITH TRICEPS EXTENSION

The wide squats with triceps extension works your glutes, your inner and outer thighs, and the backs of your arms.

TECHNIQUE AND FORM

1 Take a wide stance (legs more than a few feet apart). Bend your legs, pressing your knees to the side.

2 With both hands, hold one weight behind your head, your arms bent at your elbows.

3 Exhale and pull your abdominals in toward your spine as you straighten your legs. Extend your arms up over your head, pressing the weight toward the ceiling.

4 Hold the top position for a couple of seconds.

5 Lower to start position.

TRAINER'S TIPS

When extending your arms, keep your elbows in by your head and facing front (not out to the side).

Keep a slight bend in your knees and in your arms, even as you straighten. You don't want to lock out your joints.

WIDE SQUATS WITH TRICEPS EXTENSION

KNEE-UP INTO BACK LUNGE WITH BICEP CURL

This one's like a caffeine rush! Your heart will pump, your legs will feel strong, and your arms will get a great workout. This is a very advanced exercise, so work up to it by performing the lunge/bicep curl without weights until you have good balance.

TECHNIQUE AND FORM

1 Stand straight, with your knees slightly bent and a natural curve to your spine. Hold a weight in each hand by your sides.

2 Exhale as you bring your right knee up in front of you and start to perform alternating biceps curls, beginning with your left arm.

3 Bring your right knee back down and behind your body, so that you are performing a back lunge with your right leg. Bring the knee close to the floor when you lunge.

4 Perform the desired number of reps with the right leg, then switch to the left leg and perform the desired number of reps.

TRAINER'S TIPS

To modify this exercise, if you are a beginner you can perform it without weights or alternate from right to left leg instead of performing consecutive reps with the same leading leg.

Balance is important in this exercise. Use your core to pull your abs in tight as you lift your knee up. Ground yourself with your standing leg concentrate on pressing through the heel of your standing leg to give you support.

KNEE-UP INTO BACK LUNGE WITH BICEP CURL

UPRIGHT ROW WITH SIDE-TO-SIDE LUNGES

A great muscle builder for your upper back and legs, this fast moving exercise has cardio benefits too!

TECHNIQUE AND FORM

1 Stand with your knees slightly bent, a weight in each hand at the front of your thighs, with your palms turned in toward your body.

2 Lunge to your right, with your right leg leading. At the same time as you lunge, bring the weights up to your chest in an upward rowing motion (elbows out to the side).

3 Come out of the lunge, turn to your left and lunge to your left. At the same time as you lunge, bring the weights up to your chest in an upward rowing motion (elbows out to the side).

TRAINER'S TIPS

Keep your elbows slightly above the weights as you perform the row.

Lift the weights only as high as your chest or you could injure your shoulders.

UPRIGHT ROW WITH SIDE-TO-SIDE LUNGES

SQUAT WITH ALTERNATING LEG KICK

Control is essential in this great exercise for the heart and legs muscles. Never kick wildly.

TECHNIQUE AND FORM

1 Stand straight, with your knees slightly bent and a slight curve to your spine and your feet approximately shoulder width apart. Hold a dumbbell in each hand; keep your arms down by your sides.

2 Inhale and lower into the squat position with your knees bent, your hips pressed out behind you, and your thighs going no lower than parallel to the floor.

3 Exhale as you straighten your legs; once they are almost straight press your left leg out to the side.

4 As you bring your left leg down, immediately perform a squat.

5 Repeat, this time pressing your right leg out to the side as you come out of the squat.

TRAINER'S TIPS

Think about pressing your leg rather than kicking it this will help you to use less momentum and more muscle.

You don't have to lift your leg up high to get benefits from this exercise. Lift high enough so that you feel a tightening in your outer thighs, but never any sharp pain.

To increase intensity of this exercise you can perform side arm raises with dumbbells as you come out of the squat.

SQUAT WITH ALTERNATING LEG KICK

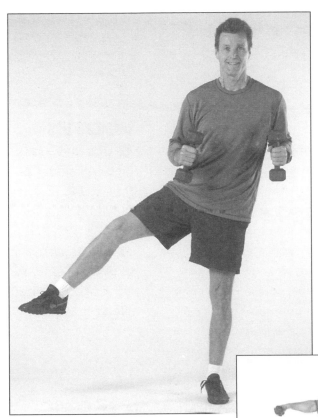

VARIATION

PUSH-UP WITH SIDE ROTATION

A toughie, this exercise requires significant core (ab/back) strength. Work up to it.

TECHNIQUE AND FORM

1   Face the floor in a push-up-ready position with your arms extended and wider than your chest and your back flat.

2   Bend your arms and lower your chest so that it hovers a couple of inches above the floor.

3   Push back up as you exhale.

4   When you reach the top, lift your right arm off the floor and rotate your body so that you are balancing on your left arm and left foot.

5   Rotate back and return your right hand to the floor. Lower your chest again.

6   Push back up as you exhale this time lifting your left arm off the floor and rotating your body so that you are balancing on your right side.

TRAINER'S TIPS

✪   To work up to this exercise, begin by performing regular push-ups on bent knees. Progress to performing push-ups with straight legs before adding the rotation.

✪   Think about using your abs and lower back muscles to stabilize your body as you lift. Also think about grounding your body with the opposite arm and leg.

PUSH-UP WITH SIDE ROTATION

DEADLIFT/ ROW COMBO

Perform this exercise for your hamstrings, lower and mid-back.

TECHNIQUE AND FORM

1 Stand straight with a weight in each hand.

2 Keeping your back nearly straight, bend at your hips so that the weights are just below your knees. Your palms should face to the rear.

3 Exhale and straighten. As you do so, bring the weights in toward your navel, pulling your elbows behind your back to perform a row.

TRAINER'S TIPS

Proper form is vital to avoid injury to the lower back. Never curve your back when you bend forward. Pulling in your abs tightly can help you to maintain proper form.

Only go as low as you can in good form.

When you perform the row, concentrate on squeezing the back muscles for a second or two.

To protect your wrists, you can perform this exercise with a barbell.

DEADLIFT/ ROW COMBO

VARIATION

Chapter 9
Machine Exercises

As we've mentioned, we prefer that you use dumbbells for your 21-Minute *EXPRESS* Workout whenever possible because of the increased amount of neuromuscular stimulation free weight-based workouts provide. That said, there are times when you may need to choose a machine-based workout—for example, if you are away and your hotel gym has no free weights. There are also times when a machine workout is preferable to a dumbbell version—such as when you have an injury or muscular weakness and you need the extra support a machine provides.

This chapter presents all the machine-based exercises for the *EXPRESS* Workout. The most important thing is to make sure you have proper form and the machine is on the correct settings for your height and fitness level. Since positions vary depending on machine and manufacturer, carefully read the position instructions that are nearly always posted on the machine.

THE**BODY**
SCULPTING
BIBLE
EXPRESS

9

TWO-ARM ROW MACHINE
BACK AND CHEST

This machine targets the mid-back muscles along with the latissimus dorsi. Secondary emphasis is placed on the trapezius, rhomboids and biceps brachii muscles. For a similar dumbbell exercise, try the One-Arm Row with either grip.

TECHNIQUE AND FORM

1 Sit on the machine and position your chest against the pad. Depending on the machine used, you may need to adjust the length of the chest pad and the height of the seat in a manner that allows your arms to be perpendicular to your torso (at a 90 degree angle) when you grasp the handle bars.

2 Select the desired resistance and grasp the handle bars with a neutral grip (palms facing each other and thumb pointing towards the ceiling). Your arms should be extended in front of you and your shoulders should be stretched. This will be your starting position.

3 Using your back muscles and not your arms, pull the machine lever back towards you until your elbows are past your back and shoulders are pulled back. Hold the contracted position for a second. Breathe out as you perform this movement.

TRAINER'S TIPS

It is important that you adjust the machine so that your arms at a 90 degree angle from your torso so that back muscle stimulation is maximized. If the arms are too high then the biceps will take the brunt of the work.

Keep control of the machine at all times and concentrate on using the back muscles as opposed to the arms.

The movement can also be performed with a palms down grip or a palms up grip as well. This just slightly changes the angle of stimulation.

©2004 Blue Star Creative

BENCH PRESS MACHINE
BACK AND CHEST

This machine targets the pectoralis major (the mid chest portion). Secondary emphasis is placed on the clavicular portion of the pectoralis major (upper chest), anterior deltoids and triceps. Two dumbbell exercises similar to this machine are the Flat Dumbbell Bench Press and the Incline Dumbbell Bench Press.

TECHNIQUE AND FORM

1 Sit on the machine and adjust the seat of the machine so that your upper chest is placed just above the handle bars provided by the lever.

2 Select the desired resistance and grasp the handle bars with an overhand grip (palms facing down and thumbs pointing towards each other). Your elbows should be placed out to the sides. The torso, shoulders and upper arms should be elevated, creating a 90 degree angle between the torso and the upper arms. There should be a straight imaginary line between the bottom of the neck and the elbow. (Note: Most of these machines have a foot lever that allows for the upper lever to come forward so that you can grasp it. If this is the case, then you will need to push the foot lever so that you can grasp the handle bars.)

3 Using your chest muscles and not your arms, push the machine lever away from you until your arms are fully extended in front of you. Hold the contracted position for a second. Breathe out as you perform this movement.

4 Return to the starting position as you inhale.

TRAINER'S TIPS

The only body parts moving should be the arms as they move the lever forward. The back and head should always remain on the seat. Many people bring the head forward as they perform the movement but this can hyperextend the neck muscles.

Keep control of the machine at all times and concentrate on using the chest muscles as opposed to the arms.

WIDE GRIP PULLDOWNS TO FRONT

BACK AND CHEST

This machine targets the latissimus dorsi. Secondary emphasis is placed on the mid-back muscles, trapezius, rhomboids and biceps brachii muscles. For a similar dumbbell exercise, try the One-Arm Row with either hand grip.

©2004 Nautilus, Inc., The Nautilus Group

TECHNIQUE AND FORM

1 Select the desired resistance and adjust the height of the thigh supports that prevent the body weight from moving up.

2 Grasp the wide bar on the overhead pulley with an overhand grip (palms facing down) about 3 inches away from shoulder width.

3 As you have both arms extended in front of you holding the bar at the chosen grip width, bring your torso back around 30 degrees or so while creating a curvature on your lower back and sticking your chest out. This is your starting position.

4 As you breathe out, pull the bar down until it touches your upper chest by drawing the shoulders and the upper arms down and back. Concentrate on squeezing the back muscles once you reach the fully contracted position and keep the elbows close to your body. The upper torso should remain stationary as your bring the bar to you and only the arms should move. The forearms should do no other work other than hold the bar.

5 After a second on the contracted position, while breathing in, slowly bring the bar back to the starting position when your arms are fully extended and the lats are fully stretched.

TRAINER'S TIPS

⊗ The only body parts moving should be the arms as they move the pulley towards your chest. The back and head should always remain stationary avoiding any type of swinging that could be damaging to the lower back.

⊗ Ensure that the bar is taken to the upper chest and not the stomach.

PECK DECK MACHINE
BACK AND CHEST

©2004 Blue Star Creative

This machine targets the pectoralis major (the mid chest portion). Secondary emphasis is placed on the clavicular portion of the pectoralis major (upper chest), and anterior deltoids.

TECHNIQUE AND FORM

1 Sit on the machine and adjust the seat so that your upper chest is placed just above the handle bars provided by the lever.

2 Select the desired resistance and grasp the handle bars with a neutral grip (palms facing each other).

3 Position your upper arms in front of you, hands close to each other and upper arms parallel to the floor. This will be your starting position.

4 Move the levers back to the stretched position in which the arms will be in line with your torso (with a straight line between the bottom of the neck and the elbows). Breathe in as you perform this movement.

5 Bring the levers back to the starting position as you exhale and contract the chest muscles. Hold for a second.

TRAINER'S TIPS

Keep a slight bend to your elbows in order to prevent stress at the biceps tendon.

Keep your back and head on the back pad as moving it forward can put undue stress on the neck.

Some machines have pads instead of handles. If this is the case, then the same movement is performed but you'll need to bend at the elbows at a 90 degree angle with your upper arms parallel to floor and place your forearms on the padded lever.

125

BICEPS CURL MACHINE
ARMS

This movement targets the biceps brachii with secondary emphasis on the brachialis. A dumbbell exercise similar to this machine is the Dumbbell Curls.

TECHNIQUE AND FORM

1 Adjust the seat of the machine so that your upper chest is placed just above the arm pad provided by the machine.

2 Grasp the handles with an underhand grip and position the elbows on top of the arm pad at shoulder width distance. This will be your starting position.

3 Raise the handle bars as you breathe out until the biceps are fully flexed with the back of the upper arm remaining on the pad.

4 Return to the starting position as you inhale.

TRAINER'S TIPS

✪ Keep the elbows always in contact with the pad. This will ensure full biceps stimulation.

✪ The upper body should remain stationary.

TRICEPS EXTENSION MACHINE
ARMS

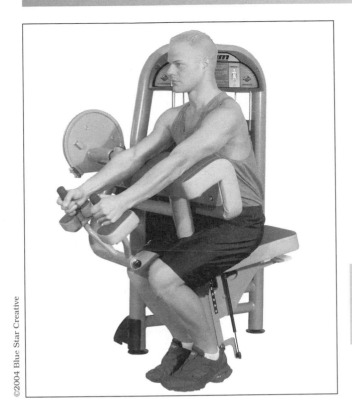

©2004 Blue Star Creative

This movement targets the triceps brachii. A similar dumbbell exercise is the Lying Dumbbell Triceps Extension.

TECHNIQUE AND FORM

1 Sit on the machine and adjust the seat of the machine so that your upper chest is placed just above the arm pad provided by the machine.

2 Grasp the handles with a neutral grip (palms facing each other) and position the elbows on top of the arm pad at shoulder width distance. This will be your starting position.

3 Push the lever down until the arm is fully extended. Breathe out as you perform this movement.

4 Return to the starting position as you breathe in.

TRAINER'S TIPS

✖ Keep the elbows always in contact with the pad. This will ensure full triceps stimulation.

✖ The upper body should remain stationary.

HIGH PULLEY CABLE CURLS ON PULLDOWN MACHINE

This movement targets the biceps brachii with secondary emphasis on the brachialis. A similar dumbbell exercise is the Dumbbell Curls.

TECHNIQUE AND FORM

❶ Stand in front of a pulldown machine with a bar attached to the pulley. If the machine has a bench, simply straddle it.

❷ Grab the bar using a shoulder wide grip and position your upper arms in a way that they are parallel to the floor with the palms of the hands facing up. This will be your starting position.

❸ Curl the bar towards you until it is close to your forehead. Make sure that as you do so you flex your biceps and exhale. The upper arms should remain stationary and only the forearms should move. Hold for a second on the contracted position.

❹ Slowly bring back the arms to the starting position as you inhale.

TRAINER'S TIPS

✪ When you grab the bar before starting the exercise you may slant your torso a bit backwards to maintain good balance.

✪ It is of utmost importance that the upper arms remain stationary as moving them will take off stimulation from the biceps.

TRICEPS PUSHDOWNS
ARMS

©2004 Blue Star Creative

This movement targets the triceps brachii. A simliar dumbbell exercise is the Lying Dumbbell Triceps Extension.

TECHNIQUE AND FORM

1 Sit on machine. Grasp handles with your palms facing inward. this is your starting position.

2 Lower the handles until your arms are extended. Your upper arms should remain stationary next to your torso. only your forearms move. Exhale as you perform this movement.

3 Hold at the contraction position. Then, slowly bring the handles back up to the starting position. Breathe in as you perform this step.

TRAINER'S TIPS

It is of utmost importance that the upper arms remain stationary next to your torso as moving them will take off stimulation from the triceps.

SHOULDER PRESS MACHINE
SHOULDERS AND CALVES

This movement targets the same muscles used on a Dumbbell Shoulder Press movement with less activation of muscle fibers as there is no need to balance the weights.

TECHNIQUE AND FORM

1 Adjust the seat of the machine to your height.

2 Select a weight and grasp the handles.

3 As you exhale, push the machine lever up until your arms are fully extended.

4 After a second pause, slowly come down back to the starting position as you inhale.

TRAINER'S TIPS

✪ Keep the wrist straight and avoid the temptation of bending it backwards as that places undue strain on it.

CALF RAISE MACHINE

This movement also targets the gastrocnemius muscle in the calves. Similar dumbbell exercises include the One- and Two-Legged Calf Raise.

TECHNIQUE AND FORM

1 Adjust the padded lever of the calf raise machine to fit your height.

2 Place your shoulders under the pads provided and position your toes facing forward, inward, or outward. The balls of your feet should be secured on top of the calf block with the heels extending off it. Push the lever up by extending your hips and knees until your torso is standing erect. The knees should be kept with a slight bend and never be locked. Toes should be facing forward. This will be your starting position.

3 Raise your heels as you breathe out by extending your ankles as high as possible and flexing your calf. Ensure that the knee is kept stationary at all times. There should be no bending at any time. Hold the contracted position by a second before you start to go back down.

4 Go back slowly to the starting position as you breathe in by lowering your heels as you bend the ankles until calves are stretched.

TRAINER'S TIPS

⚹ If you suffer from lower back problems, a better exercise is the calf press as during a standing calf raise the back has to support the weight being lifted.

⚹ Maintain your back straight and stationary at all times. Rounding of the back can cause lower back injury.

REVERSE FLY MACHINE
SHOULDERS AND CALVES

This machine targets the rear deltoid most effectively. This is one of the few machines which is almost as effective as its free weight version, the Bent-Over Lateral Raise, due to the degree of isolation that it provides.

©2004 Blue Star Creative

TECHNIQUE AND FORM

1 Adjust the seat so that the handles are at shoulder height and sit on the machine with your torso pressed against the pad.

2 Grasp the handles.

3 Slightly bend your elbows and rotate your shoulders so that the elbows are to the sides. This is your starting position.

4 Using your rear deltoid muscles, pull the levers apart and to the rear until elbows are just behind your back. There should be a slight bend at the elbows. Exhale as you perform this movement and hold the contraction for a second.

5 Slowly return to the starting position as you inhale.

TRAINER'S TIPS

Ensure that the elbows do not drop below the shoulders in order to maximize rear deltoid involvement. If you let the elbows drop, then you start using the back muscles more to perform the movement, thus taking away from deltoid stimulation.

LYING LEG CURL MACHINE

LOWER BODY AND ABS

This is a good isolation machine for the hamstrings. A dumbbell equivalent is the Dumbbell Stiff-Legged Deadlifts.

TECHNIQUE AND FORM

1 Adjust the machine lever to fit your height and lie face down on the leg curl machine (preferably one where the pad is angled as opposed to flat since an angled position is more favorable for hamstrings recruitment) with the pad of the lever on the back of your legs (just a few inches under the calves).

2 Keeping the torso flat on the bench, ensure your legs are fully stretched and grab the side handles of the machine. Position your toes straight. This will be your starting position.

3 As you exhale, curl your legs up as far as possible without lifting the upper legs from the pad. Once you hit the fully contracted position, hold it for a second.

4 As you inhale, bring the legs back to the initial position.

TRAINER'S TIPS

Do not ever use so much weight on the exercise that you start using swinging and jerking as you can risk both lower back injury and also a hamstring tear.

LEG EXTENSION MACHINE
LOWER BODY AND ABS

This is a great machine for isolating the quadriceps muscles. Two similar dumbbell exercises are the Static Dumbbell Lunges and the Dumbbell Squats.

TECHNIQUE AND FORM

1 Sit on the machine with your legs under the pad (feet pointed forward) and hold the side bars. This will be your starting position. Note: You will need to adjust the pad so that it falls on top of your lower leg (just above your feet).

2 Using your quadriceps, extend your legs to the maximum as you exhale. Ensure that the rest of the body remains stationary on the seat. Pause a second on the contracted position.

3 Slowly lower the weight back to the original position as you inhale, ensuring that you do not go past the 90 degree angle limit.

TRAINER'S TIPS

⬧ Avoid fast jerking motion on the way up as that puts undue stress on the kneecaps.

⬧ Make sure that your legs form a 90 degree angle between the lower and upper leg. If the angle is less than 90 degrees then that means the knee is over the toes which in turn creates undue stress at the knee joint. If the machine is designed that way, either look for another machine or just make sure that when you start executing the exercise you stop going down once you hit the 90 degree angle.

©2004 Blue Star Creative

LEG PRESS MACHINE
LOWER BODY AND ABS

Good basic exercise for the legs, albeit not as effective as a squat.

TECHNIQUE AND FORM

1 Using a leg press machine, sit down on the machine and place your legs on the platform directly in front of you at a medium (shoulder width) foot stance.

2 Your torso and legs should make a 90 degree angle with your legs fully extended in front of you. (Note: Do not lock your knees.) This will be your starting position.

3 As you inhale, slowly lower yourself until your upper and lower legs make a 90 degree angle.

4 Pushing mainly with the toes and using the quadriceps, exhale and return to the starting position.

TRAINER'S TIPS

If you are using a machine that involves safety bars, exit the machine by getting your legs out first to one side and then your body. Remember to lock the safety pins properly once you are done. You do not want that platform falling on your fully loaded.

WIDE-STANCE LEG PRESS (PRESS WITH HEELS)
LOWER BODY AND ABS

This movement targets the gastrocnemius muscle which is the belly of the calves. The machine pictured on the next page is used for both the Wide-Stance Leg Press and the Calf Press exercise.

TECHNIQUE AND FORM

1 Using a leg press machine, sit down on the machine and place your legs high on the platform at a wide stance with toes pointed out at least 45 degrees out.

2 Your torso and the legs should make a 90 degree angle with your legs fully extended in front of you. (Note: Do not lock your knees.). This will be your starting position.

3 As you inhale, slowly lower yourself until your upper and lower legs bend past a 90 degree angle.

4 Pushing mainly with the heels and using the glutes and hamstrings, exhale and return to the starting position.

TRAINER'S TIPS

⊗ Do not lock out the knees at the top of the movement as this places undue stress on the knees.

⊗ Remember to push with the heel as the purpose is to stimulate the glutes/hamstring tie in on the back of the leg.

CALF PRESS
CALVES

This movement targets the gastrocnemius and soleus muscles of the calves.

TECHNIQUE AND FORM

1 Using a leg press machine, sit down on the machine and place your legs on the platform directly in front of you at a medium (shoulder width) foot stance.

2 Your torso and the legs should make a perfect 90 degree angle. Now carefully place your toes and balls of your feet on the lower portion of the platform with the heels extending off. Toes should be facing forward, outwards, or inwards. This will be your starting position.

3 Press on the platform by raising your heels as you breathe out by extending your ankles as high as possible and flexing your calf. Ensure that the knee is kept stationary at all times. There should be no bending at any time. Hold the contracted position by a second before you start to go back down.

4 Go back slowly to the starting position as you breathe in by lowering your heels as you bend the ankles until calves are stretched.

TRAINER'S TIPS

Make sure you don't use weight that is too heavy or you will strain your knees.

Part III

The Workouts

This part contains the 21-Day Challenge specially designed to jumpstart your exercise program. We also give you two six-week Express Workouts, one featuring dumbbell-only exercises and one using stack machines. You will find optional workouts that focus on your abs and cardio, and on your upper body, if you would like to work those areas even more intensively.

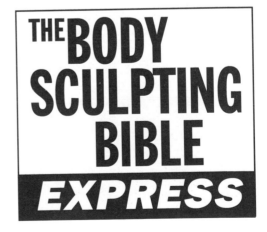

THE **BODY SCULPTING BIBLE** EXPRESS

Chapter 10
The 21-Day Challenge

THE 21-DAY GET BACK IN SHAPE BODY SCULPTING CHALLENGE!

This routine was written for two types of men: absolute beginners that have never worked out before, and those who have worked out before but have been out of the gym for a while. This routine is guaranteed to put on at least a couple of pounds of muscle and to burn at least 3 to 4 pounds of fat in 21 days, if followed together with the nutrition program recommended in the book. This challenge requires you to perform daily activities that last a maximum of 21 minutes. These activities only require a pair of adjustable dumbbells, a bench, and some sort of cardiovascular equipment.

After the 21-Day Challenge is completed, you can graduate to the less time-consuming 21-Minute *EXPRESS* Workouts that are presented in the next chapter.

Note: For best results with this program, follow the low calorie plan throughout the duration of the three-week challenge and only have 1 cheat meal on Day 21.

THE**BODY**
SCULPTING
BIBLE
EXPRESS

10

21-Day Challenge

Week 1

SPECIAL INSTRUCTIONS: Use Modified Compound Supersets. Perform Modified Compound Supersets by performing the first exercise, resting for the prescribed rest period, performing the second exercise, resting the prescribed rest period, and going back to the first one. Continue in this manner until you have performed all of the prescribed number of sets. Then continue with the next modified compound superset.

		EXERCISE	PAGE NO.	REPS	SETS	REST
WEDNESDAY						**DAY 10**
MODIFIED COMPOUND SUPERSET # 1		Back: One-Arm Row (Palms facing Torso)	52	18-20	2	60 sec
		Chest: Incline Dumbbell Bench Press	54	18-20	2	60 sec
MODIFIED COMPOUND SUPERSET # 2		Biceps: Dumbbell Curls	62	18-20	2	60 sec
		Triceps: Lying Dumbbell Triceps Extension	64	18-20	2	60 sec

		EXERCISE	PAGE NO.	REPS	SETS	REST
TUESDAY/SATURDAY						**DAY 2 AND 6**
		Lower Abs: Lying Leg Raises	90	18-20	2	60 sec
Aerobic Activity						
13 minutes of fast paced walking, stationary bike, or any other type of aerobic activity that you like.						

WEDNESDAY — DAY 3

	EXERCISE	PAGE NO.	REPS	SETS	REST
MODIFIED COMPOUND SUPERSET # 1	Thighs: Dumbbell Squats	82	18-20	2	60 sec
	Hamstrings: Static Dumbbell Lunges (Press with Heels)	84	18-20	2	60 sec
MODIFIED COMPOUND SUPERSET # 2	Calves: One-Legged Dumbbell Calf Raises	72	18-20	2	60 sec
	Shoulders: Dumbbell Shoulder Press	74	18-20	2	60 sec

THURSDAY/SUNDAY — DAY 4 AND 7

EXERCISE	PAGE NO.	REPS	SETS	REST
Upper Abs: Crunches	92	18-20	2	60 sec

Aerobic Activity
13 minutes of fast paced walking, stationary bike, or any other type of aerobic activity that you like.

FRIDAY — DAY 5

	EXERCISE	PAGE NO.	REPS	SETS	REST
MODIFIED COMPOUND SUPERSET # 1	Back: One-Arm Row (Palms facing Rear)	56	18-20	2	60 sec
	Chest: Flat Dumbbell Bench Press	58	18-20	2	60 sec
MODIFIED COMPOUND SUPERSET # 2	Biceps: Hammer Curls	66	18-20	2	60 sec
	Triceps: Overhead Dumbbell Triceps Extension	68	18-20	2	60 sec

21-Day Challenge Week 2

SPECIAL INSTRUCTIONS: Use Modified Compound Supersets. Perform Modified Compound Supersets by performing the first exercise, resting for the prescribed rest period, performing the second exercise, resting the prescribed rest period and going back to the first one. Continue in this manner until you have performed all of the prescribed number of sets. Then continue with the next modified compound superset.

MONDAY						DAY 8
		EXERCISE	**PAGE NO.**	**REPS**	**SETS**	**REST**
MODIFIED COMPOUND SUPERSET # 1		Thighs: Wide-Stance Dumbbell Squats	86	15-18	3	45 sec
		Hamstrings: Dumbbell Stiff-Legged Deadlifts	88	15-18	3	45 sec
MODIFIED COMPOUND SUPERSET # 2		Calves: Two-Legged Dumbbell Calf Raises	76	15-18	3	45 sec
		Shoulders: Bent-Over Lateral Raises	78	15-18	3	45 sec

TUESDAY/SATURDAY						DAY 9 AND 13
		EXERCISE	**PAGE NO.**	**REPS**	**SETS**	**REST**
		Lower Abs: Lying Leg Raises	90	15-18	3	45 sec
Aerobic Activity 15 minutes of fast paced walking, stationary bike, or any other type of aerobic activity that you like.						

WEDNESDAY — DAY 10

		EXERCISE	PAGE NO.	REPS	SETS	REST
MODIFIED COMPOUND SUPERSET # 1		Back: One-Arm Row (Palms facing Torso)	52	15-18	3	45 sec
		Chest: Incline Dumbbell Bench Press	54	15-18	3	45 sec
MODIFIED COMPOUND SUPERSET # 2		Biceps: Dumbbell Curls	62	15-18	3	45 sec
		Triceps: Lying Dumbbell Triceps Extension	64	15-18	3	45 sec

THURSDAY/SUNDAY — DAY 11 AND 14

		EXERCISE	PAGE NO.	REPS	SETS	REST
		Upper Abs: Crunches	92	18-20	2	60 sec

Aerobic Activity
15 minutes of fast paced walking, stationary bike, or any other type of aerobic activity that you like.

FRIDAY — DAY 12

		EXERCISE	PAGE NO.	REPS	SETS	REST
MODIFIED COMPOUND SUPERSET # 1		Thighs: Dumbbell Squats	82	15-18	3	45 sec
		Hamstrings: Static Dumbbell Lunges (Press with Heels)	84	15-18	3	45 sec
MODIFIED COMPOUND SUPERSET # 2		Calves: One-Legged Dumbbell Calf Raises	72	15-18	3	45 sec
		Shoulders: Dumbbell Shoulder Press	74	15-18	3	45 sec

21-Day Challenge   Week 3

SPECIAL INSTRUCTIONS: Use Modified Compound Supersets. Perform Modified Compound Supersets by performing the first exercise, resting for the prescribed rest period, performing the second exercise, resting the prescribed rest period and going back to the first one. Continue in this manner until you have performed all of the prescribed.

MONDAY						DAY 15
		EXERCISE	**PAGE NO.**	**REPS**	**SETS**	**REST**
MODIFIED COMPOUND SUPERSET # 1		Back: One-Arm Row (Palms facing Rear)	56	12-15	4	30 sec
		Chest: Flat Dumbbell Bench Press	58	12-15	4	30 sec
MODIFIED COMPOUND SUPERSET # 2		Biceps: Hammer Curls	66	12-15	4	30 sec
		Triceps: Overhead Dumbbell Triceps Extension	68	12-15	4	30 sec

TUESDAY/SATURDAY					DAY 16 AND 20
	EXERCISE	**PAGE NO.**	**REPS**	**SETS**	**REST**
	Lower Abs: Lying Leg Raises	90	12-15	4	30 sec

Aerobic Activity
18 minutes of fast paced walking, stationary bike, or any other type of aerobic activity that you like.

WEDNESDAY — DAY 17

		EXERCISE	PAGE NO.	REPS	SETS	REST
MODIFIED COMPOUND SUPERSET # 1		Thighs: Wide-Stance Dumbbell Squats	86	12-15	4	30 sec
		Hamstrings: Dumbbell Stiff-Legged Deadlifts	88	12-15	4	30 sec
MODIFIED COMPOUND SUPERSET # 2		Calves: Two-Legged Dumbbell Calf Raises	76	12-15	4	30 sec
		Shoulders: Bent-Over Lateral Raises	78	12-15	4	30 sec

THURSDAY/SUNDAY — DAY 18 AND 21

	EXERCISE	PAGE NO.	REPS	SETS	REST
	Upper Abs: Crunches	92	12-15	4	30 sec

Aerobic Activity
18 minutes of fast paced walking, stationary bike, or any other type of aerobic activity that you like.

WEDNESDAY — DAY 19

		EXERCISE	PAGE NO.	REPS	SETS	REST
MODIFIED COMPOUND SUPERSET # 1		Back: One-Arm Row (Palms facing Torso)	52	12-15	4	30 sec
		Chest: Incline Dumbbell Bench Press	54	12-15	4	30 sec
MODIFIED COMPOUND SUPERSET # 2		Biceps: Dumbbell Curls	62	12-15	4	30 sec
		Triceps: Lying Dumbbell Triceps Extension	64	12-15	4	30 sec

Chapter 11
The *EXPRESS* Workouts

The Body Sculpting Bible *EXPRESS* program offers three workouts. One is the all-dumbbell workout that can be performed either in the comfort of your home, or at a gym, with an adjustable bench and a set of dumbbells. The second workout is one that makes use of selectorized weight machine equipment (or weight stack machines). This is a good workout to use while on vacation at a hotel gym that does not offer dumbbells.

These workouts are designed to be done three days each week within a 21-minute limit. They are fast-paced, providing good cardiovascular conditioning as well as toning and strengthening. On the days off you can perform some abdominal work in the comfort of your home along with some optional cardiovascular exercise. For the fastest results, you are encouraged to use the dumbbell workout in addition to adding the optional cardiovascular exercise component on your days off.

THE BODY SCULPTING BIBLE EXPRESS

11

MONDAY	TUESDAY	WEDNESDAY	THURSDAY	FRIDAY	SATURDAY	SUNDAY
Day 1	Abs/Cardio	Day 2	Abs/Cardio	Day 3	Abs/Cardio	Off
Day 1	Abs/Cardio	Day 2	Abs/Cardio	Day 3	Abs/Cardio	Off

Three days a week weight training with three different routines each week.
Three days of abdominals with optional cardiovascular exercise.

Workout #1: Dumbbell Only

SPECIAL INSTRUCTIONS: Use Modified Compound Supersets. Perform Modified Compound Supersets by performing the exercises and resting the prescribed rest period until you have completed a circuit. Then, start at the beginning and repeat for the recommended number of times before moving on to the next superset.

ABS AND CARDIO				
EXERCISE	**PAGE NO.**	**REPS**	**SETS**	**REST**
MODIFIED COMPOUND SUPERSET # 1				
Lower Abs: Lying Leg Raises	90	12-15	2	30 seconds
Upper Abs: Crunches	92	12-15	2	30 seconds
Aerobic Activity				
15 minutes of fast paced walking, stationary bike, or any other type of aerobic activity that you like.				

DAY 1				
EXERCISE	**PAGE NO.**	**REPS**	**SETS**	**REST**
MODIFIED COMPOUND SUPERSET # 1				
Back: One-Arm Row (Palms facing Torso)	52	12-15	2	30 seconds
Chest: Incline Dumbbell Bench Press	54	12-15	2	30 seconds
Back: One-Arm Row (Palms facing Rear)	56	12-15	2	30 seconds
Chest: Flat Dumbbell Bench Press	58	12-15	2	30 seconds
MODIFIED COMPOUND SUPERSET # 2				
Biceps: Dumbbell Curls	62	12-15	2	30 seconds
Triceps: Lying Dumbbell Triceps Extension	64	12-15	2	30 seconds
Biceps: Hammer Curls	66	12-15	2	30 seconds
Triceps: Overhead Dumbbell Triceps Extension	68	12-15	2	30 seconds

Weeks 1 & 2

DAY 2

EXERCISE	PAGE NO.	REPS	SETS	REST
MODIFIED COMPOUND SUPERSET # 1				
Thighs: Dumbbell Squats	82	12-15	2	30 seconds
Hamstrings: Static Dumbbell Lunges (Press with Heels)	84	12-15	2	30 seconds
Thighs: Wide-Stance Dumbbell Squats	86	12-15	2	30 seconds
Hamstrings: Dumbbell Stiff-Legged Deadlifts	88	12-15	2	30 seconds
MODIFIED COMPOUND SUPERSET # 2				
Calves: One-Legged Dumbbell Calf Raises	72	12-15	2	30 seconds
Shoulders: Dumbbell Shoulder Press	74	12-15	2	30 seconds
Calves: Two-Legged Dumbbell Calf Raises	76	12-15	2	30 seconds
Shoulders: Bent-Over Lateral Raises	78	12-15	2	30 seconds

DAY 3

EXERCISE	PAGE NO.	REPS	SETS	REST
FULL BODY COMBINATION WORKOUT # 1				
Back and Thighs: Squats with Dumbbell Rows	104	12-15	2	30 seconds
Chest and Core: Push-Up with Side Rotation	116	12-15	2	30 seconds
Shoulders and Thighs: Upright Row with Side-to-Side Lunges	112	12-15	2	30 seconds
Hamstrings and Back: Deadlift/Row Combo	118	12-15	2	30 seconds
FULL BODY COMBINATION WORKOUT # 2				
Biceps and Thighs: Knee-Up into Back Lunge with Bicep Curl	110	12-15	2	30 seconds
Triceps and Thighs: Wide Squats with Triceps Extension	108	12-15	2	30 seconds
Shoulders and Thighs: Lunges with Overhead Press	106	12-15	2	30 seconds
Thighs: Squat with Alternating Leg Kick	114	12-15	2	30 seconds

Workout #1: Dumbbell Only

SPECIAL INSTRUCTIONS: Use Modified Compound Supersets. Perform two exercises without resting; rest for 30 seconds and then perform the next two exercises without resting. Rest for 30 seconds and repeat the circuit for the indicated number of sets. Then continue with the next modified compound superset.

ABS AND CARDIO

EXERCISE	PAGE NO.	REPS	SETS	REST
MODIFIED COMPOUND SUPERSET # 1				
Lower Abs: Lying Leg Raises	90	10-12	3	0 seconds
Upper Abs: Crunches	92	10-12	3	0 seconds
Aerobic Activity				
15 minutes of fast paced walking, stationary bike, or any other type of aerobic activity that you like.				

DAY 1

EXERCISE	PAGE NO.	REPS	SETS	REST
MODIFIED COMPOUND SUPERSET # 1				
Back: One-Arm Row (Palms facing Torso)	52	10-12	3	0 seconds
Chest: Incline Dumbbell Bench Press	54	10-12	3	30 seconds
Back: One-Arm Row (Palms facing Rear)	56	10-12	3	0 seconds
Chest: Flat Dumbbell Bench Press	58	10-12	3	30 seconds
MODIFIED COMPOUND SUPERSET # 2				
Biceps: Dumbbell Curls	62	10-12	3	0 seconds
Triceps: Lying Dumbbell Triceps Extension	64	10-12	3	30 seconds
Biceps: Hammer Curls	66	10-12	3	0 seconds
Triceps: Overhead Dumbbell Triceps Extension	68	10-12	3	30 seconds

Weeks 3 & 4

DAY 2

EXERCISE	PAGE NO.	REPS	SETS	REST
MODIFIED COMPOUND SUPERSET # 1				
Thighs: Dumbbell Squats	82	10-12	3	0 seconds
Hamstrings: Static Dumbbell Lunges (Press with Heels)	84	10-12	3	30 seconds
Thighs: Wide-Stance Dumbbell Squats	86	10-12	3	0 seconds
Hamstrings: Dumbbell Stiff-Legged Deadlifts	88	10-12	3	30 seconds
MODIFIED COMPOUND SUPERSET # 2				
Calves: One-Legged Dumbbell Calf Raises	72	10-12	3	0 seconds
Shoulders: Dumbbell Shoulder Press	74	10-12	3	30 seconds
Calves: Two-Legged Dumbbell Calf Raises	76	10-12	3	0 seconds
Shoulders: Bent-Over Lateral Raises	78	10-12	3	30 seconds

DAY 3

EXERCISE	PAGE NO.	REPS	SETS	REST
FULL BODY COMBINATION WORKOUT # 1				
Back and Thighs: Squats with Dumbbell Rows	104	10-12	3	0 seconds
Chest and Core: Push-Up with Side Rotation	116	10-12	3	30 seconds
Shoulders and Thighs: Upright Row with Side-to-Side Lunges	112	10-12	3	0 seconds
Hamstrings and Back: Deadlift/Row Combo	118	10-12	3	30 seconds
FULL BODY COMBINATION WORKOUT # 2				
Biceps and Thighs: Knee-Up into Back Lunge with Bicep Curl	110	10-12	3	0 seconds
Triceps and Thighs: Wide Squats with Triceps Extension	108	10-12	3	30 seconds
Shoulders and Thighs: Lunges with Overhead Press	106	10-12	3	0 seconds
Thighs: Squat with Alternating Leg Kick	114	10-12	3	30 seconds

Workout #1: Dumbbell Only

SPECIAL INSTRUCTIONS: Use Giant Sets. Perform four exercises with no rest period in between. Only rest after the four exercises have been performed consecutively. Repeat for the prescribed number of sets and then continue with the next group of exercises.

ABS AND CARDIO

EXERCISE	PAGE NO.	REPS	SETS	REST
MODIFIED COMPOUND SUPERSET # 1				
Lower Abs: Lying Leg Raises	90	8-10	3	0 seconds
Upper Abs: Crunches	92	8-10	3	0 seconds
Aerobic Activity				
15 minutes of fast paced walking, stationary bike, or any other type of aerobic activity that you like. Try to burn more calories than you did in the past two weeks by increasing your pace or intensity.				

DAY 1

EXERCISE	PAGE NO.	REPS	SETS	REST
GIANT SET # 1				
Back: One-Arm Row (Palms facing Torso)	52	8-10	3	0 seconds
Chest: Incline Dumbbell Bench Press	54	8-10	3	0 seconds
Back: One-Arm Row (Palms facing Rear)	56	8-10	3	0 seconds
Chest: Flat Dumbbell Bench Press	58	8-10	3	30 seconds
GIANT SET # 2				
Biceps: Dumbbell Curls	62	8-10	3	0 seconds
Triceps: Lying Dumbbell Triceps Extension	64	8-10	3	0 seconds
Biceps: Hammer Curls	66	8-10	3	0 seconds
Triceps: Overhead Dumbbell Triceps Extension	68	8-10	3	30 seconds

Weeks 5 & 6

DAY 2

EXERCISE	PAGE NO.	REPS	SETS	REST
GIANT SET # 1				
Thighs: Dumbbell Squats	82	8-10	3	0 seconds
Hamstrings: Static Dumbbell Lunges (Press with Heels)	84	8-10	3	0 seconds
Thighs: Wide-Stance Dumbbell Squats	86	8-10	3	0 seconds
Hamstrings: Dumbbell Stiff-Legged Deadlifts	88	8-10	3	30 seconds
GIANT SET # 2				
Calves: One-Legged Dumbbell Calf Raises	72	8-10	3	0 seconds
Shoulders: Dumbbell Shoulder Press	74	8-10	3	0 seconds
Calves: Two-Legged Dumbbell Calf Raises	76	8-10	3	0 seconds
Shoulders: Bent-Over Lateral Raises	78	8-10	3	30 seconds

DAY 3

EXERCISE	PAGE NO.	REPS	SETS	REST
FULL BODY COMBINATION GIANT SET # 1 (Heavier Weights)				
Back and Thighs: Squats with Dumbbell Rows	104	8-10	3	0 seconds
Chest and Core: Push-Up with Side Rotation	116	8-10	3	0 seconds
Shoulders and Thighs: Upright Row with Side-to-Side Lunges	112	8-10	3	0 seconds
Hamstrings and Back: Deadlift/Row Combo	118	8-10	3	30 seconds
FULL BODY COMBINATION GIANT SET # 2 (Heavier Weights)				
Biceps and Thighs: Knee-Up into Back Lunge with Bicep Curl	110	8-10	3	0 seconds
Triceps and Thighs: Wide Squats with Triceps Extension	108	8-10	3	0 seconds
Shoulders and Thighs: Lunges with Overhead Press	106	8-10	3	0 seconds
Thighs: Squat with Alternating Leg Kick	114	8-10	3	30 seconds

Workout #2: Machine Only

SPECIAL INSTRUCTIONS: Use Modified Compound Supersets. Perform Modified Compound Supersets by performing the exercises and resting the prescribed rest period until you have completed a circuit. Then, start at the beginning and repeat for the recommended number of times before moving on to the next superset.

ABS AND CARDIO

EXERCISE	PAGE NO.	REPS	SETS	REST
MODIFIED COMPOUND SUPERSET # 1				
Lower Abs: Lying Leg Raises	90	12-15	2	30 seconds
Upper Abs: Crunches	92	12-15	2	30 seconds
Aerobic Activity				
15 minutes of fast paced walking, stationary bike, or any other type of aerobic activity that you like.				

DAY 1

EXERCISE	PAGE NO.	REPS	SETS	REST
MODIFIED COMPOUND SUPERSET # 1				
Back: Two-Arm Row Machine	122	12-15	2	30 seconds
Chest: Bench Press Machine	123	12-15	2	30 seconds
Back: Wide Grip Pulldowns to Front	124	12-15	2	30 seconds
Chest: Peck Deck Machine	125	12-15	2	30 seconds
MODIFIED COMPOUND SUPERSET # 2				
Biceps: Biceps Curl Machine	126	12-15	2	30 seconds
Triceps: Triceps Extension Machine	127	12-15	2	30 seconds
Biceps: High Pulley Cable Curls on Pulldown Machine	128	12-15	2	30 seconds
Triceps: Triceps Pushdowns	129	12-15	2	30 seconds

Weeks 1 & 2

DAY 2				
EXERCISE	**PAGE NO.**	**REPS**	**SETS**	**REST**
MODIFIED COMPOUND SUPERSET # 1				
Thighs: Leg Press Machine	135	12-15	2	30 seconds
Hamstrings: Lying Leg Curl Machine	133	12-15	2	30 seconds
Thighs: Leg Extension Machine	134	12-15	2	30 seconds
Hamstrings: Wide-Stance Leg Press (Press with Heels)	136	12-15	2	30 seconds
MODIFIED COMPOUND SUPERSET # 2				
Calves: Calf Press	137	12-15	2	30 seconds
Shoulders: Shoulder Press Machine	130	12-15	2	30 seconds
Calves: Calf Raise Machine	131	12-15	2	30 seconds
Shoulders: Reverse Fly Machine	132	12-15	2	30 seconds

DAY 3				
EXERCISE	**PAGE NO.**	**REPS**	**SETS**	**REST**
FULL BODY MODIFIED COMPOUND SUPERSET # 1				
Back: Wide Grip Pulldowns to Front	124	12-15	2	30 seconds
Chest: Peck Deck Machine	125	12-15	2	30 seconds
Thighs: Leg Extension Machine	134	12-15	2	30 seconds
Hamstrings: Wide-Stance Leg Press (Press with Heels)	136	12-15	2	30 seconds
FULL BODY MODIFIED COMPOUND SUPERSET # 2				
Biceps: High Pulley Cable Curls on Pulldown Machine	128	12-15	2	30 seconds
Triceps: Triceps Pushdowns	129	12-15	2	30 seconds
Shoulders: Shoulder Press Machine	130	12-15	2	30 seconds
Calves: Calf Raise Machine	131	12-15	2	30 seconds

Workout #2: Machine Only

SPECIAL INSTRUCTIONS: Use Modified Compound Supersets. Perform two exercises without resting; rest for 30 seconds and then perform the next two exercises without resting. Rest for 30 seconds and repeat the circuit for the indicated number of sets. Then continue with the next modified compound superset.

ABS AND CARDIO

EXERCISE	PAGE NO.	REPS	SETS	REST
MODIFIED COMPOUND SUPERSET # 1				
Lower Abs: Lying Leg Raises	90	10-12	3	0 seconds
Upper Abs: Crunches	92	10-12	3	0 seconds
Aerobic Activity				
15 minutes of fast paced walking, stationary bike, or any other type of aerobic activity that you like.				

DAY 1

EXERCISE	PAGE NO.	REPS	SETS	REST
MODIFIED COMPOUND SUPERSET # 1				
Back: Two-Arm Row Machine	122	10-12	3	0 seconds
Chest: Bench Press Machine	123	10-12	3	30 seconds
Back: Wide Grip Pulldowns to Front	124	10-12	3	0 seconds
Chest: Peck Deck Machine	125	10-12	3	30 seconds
MODIFIED COMPOUND SUPERSET # 2				
Biceps: Biceps Curl Machine	126	10-12	3	0 seconds
Triceps: Triceps Extensions Machine	127	10-12	3	30 seconds
Biceps: High Pulley Cable Curls on Pulldown Machine	128	10-12	3	0 seconds
Triceps: Triceps Pushdowns	129	10-12	3	30 seconds

Weeks 3 & 4

DAY 2

EXERCISE	PAGE NO.	REPS	SETS	REST
MODIFIED COMPOUND SUPERSET # 1				
Thighs: Leg Press Machine	135	10-12	3	0 seconds
Hamstrings: Lying Leg Curl Machine	133	10-12	3	30 seconds
Thighs: Leg Extension Machine	134	10-12	3	0 seconds
Hamstrings: Wide-Stance Leg Press (Press with Heels)	136	10-12	3	30 seconds
MODIFIED COMPOUND SUPERSET # 2				
Calves: Calf Press	137	10-12	3	0 seconds
Shoulders: Shoulder Press Machine	130	10-12	3	30 seconds
Calves: Calf Raise Machine	131	10-12	3	0 seconds
Shoulders: Reverse Fly Machine	132	10-12	3	30 seconds

DAY 3

EXERCISE	PAGE NO.	REPS	SETS	REST
FULL BODY MODIFIED COMPOUND SUPERSET # 1				
Back: Wide Grip Pulldowns to Front	124	10-12	3	0 seconds
Chest: Peck Deck Machine	125	10-12	3	30 seconds
Thighs: Leg Extension Machine	134	10-12	3	0 seconds
Hamstrings: Wide-Stance Leg Press (Press with Heels)	136	10-12	3	30 seconds
FULL BODY MODIFIED COMPOUND SUPERSET # 2				
Biceps: High Pulley Cable Curls on Pulldown Machine	128	10-12	3	0 seconds
Triceps: Triceps Pushdowns	129	10-12	3	30 seconds
Shoulders: Shoulder Press Machine	130	10-12	3	0 seconds
Calves: Calf Raise Machine	131	10-12	3	30 seconds

Workout #2: Machine Only

SPECIAL INSTRUCTIONS: Use Giant Sets. Perform four exercises with no rest period in between. Only rest after the four exercises have been performed consecutively. Repeat for the prescribed number of sets and then continue with the next group of exercises.

ABS AND CARDIO

EXERCISE	PAGE NO.	REPS	SETS	REST
GIANT SET # 1				
Lower Abs: Lying Leg Raises	90	10-12	3	0 seconds
Upper Abs: Crunches	92	10-12	3	0 seconds
Obliques: Bicycle	94	12-15	2	30 seconds
Aerobic Activity				
15 minutes of fast paced walking, stationary bike, or any other type of aerobic activity that you like. Try to burn more calories than you did in the past two weeks by increasing your pace or intensity.				

DAY 1

EXERCISE	PAGE NO.	REPS	SETS	REST
GIANT SET # 1				
Back: Two-Arm Row Machine	122	10-12	3	0 seconds
Chest: Bench Press Machine	123	10-12	3	0 seconds
Thighs: Leg Press Machine	135	10-12	3	0 seconds
Hamstrings: Lying Leg Curl Machine	133	10-12	3	30 seconds
GIANT SET # 1				
Biceps: Biceps Curl Machine	126	10-12	3	0 seconds
Triceps: Triceps Extensions Machine	127	10-12	3	0 seconds
Biceps: High Pulley Cable Curls on Pulldown Machine	128	10-12	3	0 seconds
Triceps: Triceps Pushdowns	129	10-12	3	30 seconds

Weeks 5 & 6

DAY 2

EXERCISE	PAGE NO.	REPS	SETS	REST
GIANT SET # 1				
Thighs: Leg Press Machine	135	10-12	3	0 seconds
Hamstrings: Lying Leg Curl Machine	133	10-12	3	0 seconds
Thighs: Leg Extension Machine	134	10-12	3	0 seconds
Hamstrings: Wide Stance Leg Press (Press with Heels)	136	10-12	3	30 seconds
GIANT SET # 2				
Calves: Calf Press	137	10-12	3	0 seconds
Shoulders: Shoulder Press Machine	130	10-12	3	0 seconds
Calves: Calf Press	137	10-12	3	0 seconds
Triceps: Triceps Pushdowns	129	10-12	3	30 seconds

DAY 3

EXERCISE	PAGE NO.	REPS	SETS	REST
GIANT SET # 1				
Back: Wide Grip Pulldowns to Front	124	10-12	3	0 seconds
Chest: Peck Deck Machine	125	10-12	3	0 seconds
Thighs: Leg Extension Machine	134	10-12	3	0 seconds
Hamstrings: Wide-Stance Leg Press (Press with Heels)	136	10-12	3	30 seconds
GIANT SET # 2				
Biceps: High Pulley Cable Curls on Pulldown Machine	128	10-12	3	0 seconds
Triceps: Triceps Pushdowns	129	10-12	3	0 seconds
Shoulders: Reverse Fly Machine	132	10-12	3	0 seconds
Calves: Calf Raise Machine	131	10-12	3	30 seconds

Supplemental Workout

SPECIAL INSTRUCTIONS: The *EXPRESS* workout was designed to provide you with an easy to follow, challenging strength training regimen in 21 minutes. In addition, optional cardio/abs workouts are available for your off days. For those of you who may want to focus exclusively on cardio and abdominal work, you can do the following program. Once again you will work four days each week for just 21 minutes a day. You can do this program on its own or in addition to the *EXPRESS* Workout. You also can use the off days of this program to do some of the strength training routines.

WEEKS 1 AND 2

DAY 1

CARDIO: Seventeen minutes of cardiovascular exercise at an intensity that raises your heart rate into the training zone. To determine the training zone simply subtract your age from 220 and work within a range that causes your heart to beat at 60 to 80 percent of the resulting number.

ABDOMINALS/CORE

EXERCISE	PAGE NO.	REPS	SETS	REST
MODIFIED COMPOUND SUPERSET				
Lower Abs: Lying Leg Raises	90	12-15	3	15 seconds
Upper Abs: Crunches	92	12-15	3	15 seconds
Obliques: Bicycle	94	12-15	3	15 seconds
Lower Back: Extension	100	12-15	3	15 seconds

DAY 2

CARDIO: Seventeen minutes of cardiovascular exercise at an intensity that raises your heart rate into the training zone.

ABDOMINALS/CORE

EXERCISE	PAGE NO.	REPS	SETS	REST
MODIFIED COMPOUND SUPERSET				
Lower Abs: Lying Leg Raises	90	10-12	3	15 seconds
Upper Abs: Crunches	92	10-12	3	15 seconds
Obliques: Bicycle	94	10-12	3	15 seconds
Lower Back: Extension	100	10-12	3	15 seconds

Cardio/Abs Intensive

MONDAY	TUESDAY	WEDNESDAY	THURSDAY	FRIDAY	SATURDAY	SUNDAY
Day 1	Off	Day 2	Off	Day 1	Off	Day 2
Day 1	Off	Day 2	Off	Day 1	Off	Day 2

WEEKS 3 AND 4

DAY 1

CARDIO: Seventeen minutes of cardiovascular exercise at an intensity that raises your heart rate into the training zone. Try to increase the intensity over the previous two weeks by either going faster or working out against resistance (adding hills, climbs, or fast intervals).

ABDOMINALS/CORE

EXERCISE	PAGE NO.	REPS	SETS	REST
MODIFIED COMPOUND SUPERSET Lower Abs: Lying Leg Raises	90	8-10	3	0 seconds
Upper Abs: Crunches	92	8-10	3	0 seconds
Obliques: Bicycle	94	8-10	3	0 seconds
Lower Back: Extension	100	8-10	3	15 seconds

DAY 2

CARDIO: Seventeen minutes of cardiovascular exercise at an intensity that raises your heart rate into the training zone. Try to increase the intensity over the previous two weeks by either going faster or working out against resistance (adding hills, climbs, or fast intervals).

ABDOMINALS/CORE

EXERCISE	PAGE NO.	REPS	SETS	REST
MODIFIED COMPOUND SUPERSET Lower Abs: Lying Leg Raises	90	8-10	3	0 seconds
Upper Abs: Crunches	92	8-10	3	0 seconds
Obliques: Bicycle	94	8-10	3	0 seconds
Overall Core: Plank	96	3 *(hold centered for 10 seconds, left arm/right leg extended for 5 seconds, then right arm/left leg extended for 5 seconds)*	3	15 seconds

Supplemental Workout:
Cardio/Abs Intensive

WEEKS 5 AND 6

DAY 1

CARDIO: Seventeen minutes of cardiovascular exercise at an intensity that raises your heart rate into the training zone. To determine the training zone simply subtract your age from 220 and work within a range that causes your heart to beat at 60 to 80 percent of the resulting number.

ABDOMINALS/CORE

EXERCISE	PAGE NO.	REPS	SETS	REST
MODIFIED COMPOUND SUPERSET				
Lower Abs: Lying Leg Raises	90	8-10	3	0 seconds
Upper Abs: Crunches	92	8-10	3	0 seconds
Obliques: Bicycle	94	8-10	3	0 seconds
Lower Back: Extension	100	8-10	3	15 seconds

DAY 2

CARDIO: Seventeen minutes of cardiovascular exercise at an intensity that raises your heart rate into the training zone. Try speed intervals, in which you go at a very intense level for one minute and then reduce your speed for the next minute, then increase it again for a minute; continue alternating until you ve completed the 17 minutes.

ABDOMINALS/CORE

EXERCISE	PAGE NO.	REPS	SETS	REST
MODIFIED COMPOUND SUPERSET				
Lower Abs: V-Knee	98	8-10	3	0 seconds
Upper Abs: Crunches	92	8-10	3	0 seconds
Obliques: Bicycle	94	8-10	3	0 seconds
Overall Core: Plank	96	3 *(hold centered for 10 seconds, left arm/right leg extended for 5 seconds, then right arm/left leg extended for 5 seconds)*	3	15 seconds

Supplemental Workout:
Upper Body

SPECIAL INSTRUCTIONS: For those of you who really want to concentrate on building your upper body, here's a supplemental workout you can perform. This workout can be done in addition to the others in any of the other programs we presented, or in place of a lower body workout. The supersets in this workout involve performing several exercises for a single muscle group and then repeating the sequence for the desired number of sets. To increase the intensity of the workout, increase the weight you're lifting every two weeks.

SUPPLEMENTAL UPPER BODY WORKOUT

EXERCISE	PAGE NO.	REPS	SETS	REST
MODIFIED COMPOUND SUPERSET # 1				
Back: Two-Arm Row Machine	122	12-15	2	0 seconds
Back: Wide-Grip Pulldowns to Front	124	12-15	2	0 seconds
Back: One-Arm Row (Palms facing Torso)	52	12-15	2	30 seconds
MODIFIED COMPOUND SUPERSET # 2				
Chest: Incline Dumbbell Bench Press	54	12-15	2	0 seconds
Chest: Flat Dumbbell Bench Press	58	12-15	2	0 seconds
Chest: Bench Press Machine	123	12-15	2	30 seconds
MODIFIED COMPOUND SUPERSET # 3				
Shoulders: Bent-Over Lateral Raises	78	12-15	2	0 seconds
Shoulders: Reverse Fly Machine	132	12-15	2	0 seconds
Shoulders: Shoulder Press Machine	130	12-15	2	30 seconds
SET #4				
Biceps: Dumbbell Curls	62	12-15	2	30 seconds
SET #5				
Triceps: Overhead Dumbbell Triceps Extension	68	12-15	2	30 seconds

Appendix A
Training Journal

A

Research has shown that keeping a journal of your daily activity is a great way to ensure that you are meeting your exercise goals. Use the Body Sculpting Bible *EXPRESS* Training Journal to keep track of your progress.

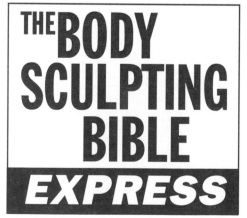

Daily Workout Journal

Week ⬤ Day ⬤

	Exercise Main (Alternate)	Rest	Set 1		Set 2		Set 3	
			Reps	Weight	Reps	Weight	Reps	Weight
Superset or Giant Set 1								
Superset or Giant Set 2								
Superset or Giant Set 1								
Superset or Giant Set 2								
Abs								

Cardio

Cardio Activity: _____   Notes: _____

Average Heart Rate: _____

Duration: _____

Use the Training Journal to keep track of your workout. Photocopy this page as many times as you need.

Appendix B

Food Charts and Nutrition

Good nutrition boils down to some simple basics:

Always try to use natural foods. Avoid using canned or prepared foods as they usually contain too much fat, sodium, and carbs.

Stay within plus or minus 10 grams of the recommended amount of carbs and proteins, plus or minus five grams for fats.

Always choose low-fat protein sources. Don't worry about incurring a fat deficiency since the supplements program takes care of the need for essential fatty acids. Besides, there are trace amounts of fats even in low-fat protein sources.

If you choose to include skim milk in your diet, remember that it not only has protein but also simple carbs. Therefore, count milk as both. Since the carbs in milk are simple carbs, this should only be used in the post workout meal. However, if you schedule requires you to include more protein shakes throughout the day, and you will rely on the carbs in skim milk, add a teaspoon of flaxseed oil to the milk to slow down the release of simple carbs into the bloodstream.

Try to include fibrous carbs in at least two meals.

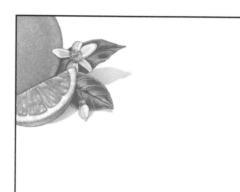

THE BODY SCULPTING BIBLE EXPRESS

B

Daily Nutrition Journal   Week ⬤ Day ⬤

	Food	Serving Size	Calories	Carbs (grams)	Protein (grams)	Fat (grams)	
Meal 1							**Meal 1**
Meal 2							**Meal 2**
Meal 3							**Meal 3**
Meal 4							**Meal 4**
Meal 5							**Meal 5**
Meal 6							**Meal 6**
TOTAL							

Use the Daily Nutrition Journal to keep track of your diet. Photocopy this page as many times as you need.

2000-Calorie Weeks

<u>Meal 1</u> (7:30 a.m.)   Breakfast (post-workout)
Choose 40 grams from Group A
Choose 40 grams from Group C

<u>Meal 2</u> (10:30 a.m.)   Morning Break Snack
Choose 40 grams from Group A
Choose 40 grams from Group B

<u>Meal 3</u> (1:30 p.m.)   Lunch Time
Choose 40 grams from Group A
Choose 30 grams from Group B
Choose 10 grams from Group D

<u>Meal 4</u> (3:30 p.m.)   Afternoon Break Snack
Choose 40 grams from Group A
Choose 40 grams from Group B

<u>Meal 5</u> (6:30 p.m.)   Dinner
Choose 40 grams from Group A
Choose 25 grams from Group B
Choose 15 grams from Group D

Note: Include one tsp of olive oil three times a day with any meals (except the post-workout meal) on one day. The next day, include one tsp of olive oil once a day and one tsp of flaxseed oil twice a day with any meals (except the post workout meal). This in conjunction with the naturally occurring fats in the food will cover your essential fats needs.

2500-Calorie Weeks

<u>Meal 1</u> (7:30 a.m.)   Breakfast (post-workout)
Choose 42 grams from Group A
Choose 42 grams from Group C

<u>Meal 2</u> (10:30 a.m.)   Morning Break Snack
Choose 42 grams from Group A
Choose 42 grams from Group B

<u>Meal 3</u> (12:30 p.m.)   Lunch Time
Choose 42 grams from Group A
Choose 30 grams from Group B
Choose 12 grams from Group D

<u>Meal 4</u> (3:30 p.m.)   Afternoon Break Snack
Choose 42 grams from Group A
Choose 42 grams from Group B

<u>Meal 5</u> (6:30 p.m.)   Dinner
Choose 42 grams from Group A
Choose 27 grams from Group B
Choose 15 grams from Group D

<u>Meal 6</u> (8:30 p.m.)   Late Snack
Choose 42 grams from Group A
Choose 22 grams from Group B
Choose 20 grams from Group D

Note: Include one tsp of olive oil three times a day with any meals (except the post workout meal) on one day. The next day, include one tsp of olive oil once a day and one tsp of flaxseed oil twice a day with any meals (except the post workout meal). This in conjunction with the naturally occurring fats in the food will cover your essential fats needs.

FOOD GROUP TABLES

For the post-workout meal, choose one item from Group A and one item from Group C in order to create a balanced meal. For all other meals, choose one item from Group A, one item from Group B, and one item from Group D. Remember to adjust the serving size depending upon the amount of nutrients that you require per meal.

GROUP A - PROTEIN			
FOOD	GRAMS	FOOD	GRAMS
Chicken breast (3.5 oz broiled)	33	White fish (3.5 oz broiled)	31
Tuna (packed in water, 3.5 oz)	35	Halibut (3.5 oz broiled)	31
Turkey breast (3.5 oz broiled)	28	Cod (3.5 oz broiled)	31
Whey protein powder (2 scoops)	22	Round steak (3.5 oz broiled)	33
10 egg whites	35	Top sirloin (4 oz)	35

Note: These weights are for uncooked portions

GROUP B - CARBOHYDRATE (COMPLEX, STARCHY)			
FOOD	GRAMS	FOOD	GRAMS
Baked potato (3.5 oz broiled)	21	Lentils (1 cup dry, cooked)	38
Plain oatmeal (1/2 cup dry)	27	Grits (1/4 cup dry)	31
Whole wheat bread (1 slice; limit if reducing body fat)	13	Pita bread (1 piece)	33
Cream of rice (1/4 cup dry, post workout only)	38	Sweet potato (4 oz)	28
Chickpeas (1 cup cooked)	45	Brown rice (2/3 cup cooked)	30

GROUP C - CARBOHYDRATE (SIMPLE)			
FOOD	GRAMS	FOOD	GRAMS
Apple (1)	15	Banana (6 oz, *post workout only*)	27
Cantaloupe (1/2)	25	Grapes (1 cup, *post workout only*)	14
Strawberries (1 cup)	9	Grapefruit (1/2)	12
Orange (1)	15	Tangerine (1)	9
Pear (1)	27	Cherries (1 cup)	22
Lemon (1)	5	Nectarine (1)	16
Peach (1)	10	Skim milk (1 cup, *preferably post workout only*)	13

GROUP D - CARBOHYDRATE (COMPLEX, FIBROUS)			
FOOD (10 OZ SERVING)	GRAMS	FOOD (10 OZ SERVING)	GRAMS
Asparagus	5	Yellow squash	12
Broccoli	17	Green beans	23
Cabbage	6	Cauliflower	12
Celery	6	Cucumber	7
Mushrooms	6	Lettuce	7
Red or Green peppers	15	Tomato	5
Spinach	3	Zucchini	13

Appendix C
Useful Resources

www.BodySculptingBible.com

A powerful resource for anyone seeking advice knowledge and more. Loaded with news, fitness tips, and discussion forums, this is a must see.

www.HRFit.net

A visit here will reward you with a well-rounded bushel of information written by Hugo Rivera, ranging from how to design a workout routine to how to select or reject a food supplement.

www.Bodybuilding.com

Tons of free information on anything you need to know about bodybuilding and fitness written by several experts in the industry. They also carry most supplement brands in the market selling them at a huge discount.

www.PowerBlocks.com

Home of the PowerBlocks™, here you will find the world's most efficient dumbbells in terms of space and feasibility of changing the weights.

www.FitnessFactory.com

A great place to fulfill your home gym equipment needs. They have awesome customer service and great prices.

www.Prolab.com

Homepage of our recommended line of supplements. They carry all of the basic supplements that bodybuilders need. In addition, all of their supplements are produced with state-of-the-art manufacturing and are sold at the right price.

www.InfinityFitness.com

Website of training and nutrition consultant Scott Mendelson. Scott is a super knowledgeable guy who has tons of free information on his site. He also carries state-of-the-art products.

www.DaveDraper.com

Dave is a bodybuilding legend. Winner of the Mr. America, Mr. World, and Mr. Universe, Dave shares his extensive knowledge in a very straightforward, simple, and almost poetic manner.

www.MuscleBuildingDiet.com

Owned by Todd Mendelsohn, a former Mr. Central Florida who works as a nutrition/training consultant. If you want more advanced tailor made programs for bulking up, this is the place to go.

Bonus Recipes *for a* Stronger *more* Sculpted Body!

A Note from Chef Marie

Following are 60 Breakfast, Lunch, Dinner and Dessert recipes. All of these recipes meet the requirements for nutritious, low-fat weight loss and, when used in conjunction with the 21-Day *EXPRESS* Body Sculpting program, are guaranteed to produce results.

How to Begin

At the start of each week, use the Daily Nutrition Journal in Appendix B to outline your meal plans. You can pick and choose your weekly meals from each category; just be sure that your daily caloric requirement is within the right range for weight loss (2000-2500).

Also, as explained on page 25, keep in mind that, during the first two weeks of your workout, you should aim to consume 2000 calories, and then increase your caloric intake to 2500 calories for the last 2 weeks. This will help your body gain muscle and lose fat more efficiently.

If you prefer to prepare your meals entirely on your own, consult the nutrition guidelines and use the food group charts in Appendix B as a guide.

A Note on Sunday Rewards

If you've stayed true to your diet all week, you deserve a reward. Treat yourself to one "cheat meal" per week. As described on pages 31-32, this can include an appetizer, main meal, and dessert. But be sure not to go overboard, or you'll run the risk of going backwards.

A Note on Times to Eat and Frequency of Meals

To help boost your metabolism, you should try to eat five or six small meals throughout the day, which amounts to approximately every 2-3 hours. This will make it easier for your body to get the energy it needs to build muscle and burn fat.

Choosing Healthier Food for Better Health

You should always try to use fresh and organic products. Limiting the amount of chemicals, colorings, preservatives, and additives in your food will benefit your body and decrease the chances of food allergies, sensitivities, and diseases.

Use canola oil, olive oil, and grapeseed oil (a great substitution to butter because of its buttery flavor) which are the healthiest fats for cooking. Those oils, plus flaxseed oil, fish oil, and walnut oil should be used for salads or cold applications. Remember that these are still fats, and you should use as little as possible which is already done in these recipes.

Reduce animal proteins and increase plant proteins such as beans or tofu. Quickly par-boil or steam vegetables to preserve their vitamins and minerals, which will also limit the addition of calories that are often found in casseroles or other vegetable dishes.

Use low-sodium and low-fat broth/stock for light sauces rather than using fats such as butter, cream, or beurre manié (butter and flour combination). Thicken sauces with cornstarch/arrowroot or waxy maze (for frozen dishes as it won't separate) instead of using flour or a flour-butter mixture. As many of these recipes are low in fat, which we know contributes to flavor, try adding flavor with fresh herbs, spices, and vegetable-concentrated broth/stock. Remember that a pinch of salt can go a long way. Way too many recipes use too much salt, which is harmful to your health because it increases blood pressure, and isn't necessary to obtain a well-balanced recipe. ■

Chef Marie-Annick Courtier is a native of Paris, France, where she learned about gourmet foods and wine in the French tradition. Chef Marie holds a Culinary Arts Degree, has worked with many world renowned chefs, and runs her own personal chef service. A Certified Fitness Nutritionist and Professional Food Manager, she also teaches cooking and created the new Certified Personal Fitness Chef Program. Chef Marie lives in Orange County, California.

One of the most important (and most commonly overlooked) aspects of a healthy diet is proper hydration. As explained on page 30, you can use the formula (0.66 x body weight) to figure out how many ounces of water you need to drink throughout the day.

Breakfast

You have probably heard the phrase "breakfast is the most important meal of the day" many times. With the hectic pace of life today, stopping to eat on your way out the door can seem like a chore. But if you don't take the time to eat first thing in the morning, you will throw off your eating regimen for the rest of the day, and risk undoing all your hard work at the gym!

Be sure to eat breakfast no later than 30 minutes after you wake up. The recipes below are designed to kickstart your day and provide you with the physical and mental energy you will need to get through the morning. Stick to it and you will notice that the first part of your day is a lot easier to handle when you provide your body with the nutrients it needs. Your energy boost is sure to increase your productivity—and encourage your metabolism to work fast, so that the pounds come off easier.

Oatmeal with Mango and Kiwi

Yield: 1 serving

 3/4 cup to 1 cup oatmeal
 1 ½ cup to 2 cups low-fat milk
 1 teaspoon almonds
 1/4 mango, diced
 1 kiwi, diced

Mix the oatmeal with the hot milk until the liquid is incorporated. Add in the almonds, mango, kiwi, and serve immediately.

Option: Add 1 ½ scoop protein powder which adds 150 calories

Per Serving (3/4 cup oatmeal): 483 Cal (18% from Fat, 16% from Protein, 66% from Carb); 21 g Protein; 10 g Tot Fat; 5 g Sat Fat; 3 g Mono Fat; 84 g Carb; 11 g Fiber; 35 g Sugar; 490 mg Calcium; 2 mg Iron; 156 mg Sodium; 29 mg Cholesterol
Per Serving (1 cup oatmeal): 611 Cal (19% from Fat, 17% from Protein, 65% from Carb); 27 g Protein; 13 g Tot Fat; 7 g Sat Fat; 4 g Mono Fat; 104 g Carb; 13 g Fiber; 41 g Sugar; 639 mg Calcium; 3 mg Iron; 206 mg Sodium; 39 mg Cholesterol

Homemade Granola with Berries

Yield: 5 to 7 servings

 1/4 cup honey
 1/4 cup vegetable oil
 1 teaspoon vanilla extract
 3 ½ cup old fashioned oats, uncooked
 1/4 cup sliced almonds
 1/4 cup pumpkin seeds
 1/4 cup raisins
 1/4 cup cranberries
 2 teaspoons cinnamon

Preheat the oven to 350°F.
 In a bowl, mix the honey, oil, vanilla extract, and cinnamon. Stir in the oats, almonds, pumpkin seeds, raisins, and cranberries. Mix well and spread over a greased cookie sheet. Bake for 10 minutes. Stir and continue to bake for another 10 minutes or until golden brown. Cool completely and break apart.

Option: Add 1 ½ scoop protein powder which adds 150 calories

Per Serving (1 serving = 3/4 cup homemade granola, 3/4 cup low-fat milk, 1/4 cup mixed fresh berries, and 1 teaspoon freshly grinded flaxseeds): 604 Cal (30% from Fat, 14% from Protein, 56% from Carb); 22 g Protein; 20 g Tot Fat; 5 g Sat Fat; 6 g Mono Fat; 87 g Carb; 13 g Fiber; 28 g Sugar; 295 mg Calcium; 5 mg Iron; 80 mg Sodium; 15 mg Cholesterol (3/4 cup homemade granola)
Per Serving (1 serving = 1 cup homemade granola, 1 cup low-fat milk, 1/4 cup mixed fresh berries, and 1 teaspoon freshly grinded flaxseeds): 832 Cal (29% from Fat, 14% from Protein, 57% from Carb); 30 g Protein; 28 g Tot Fat; 6 g Sat Fat; 8 g Mono Fat; 121 g Carb; 18 g Fiber; 38 g Sugar; 397 mg Calcium; 7 mg Iron; 107 mg Sodium; 20 mg Cholesterol (1 cup homemade granola)

Kashi Flakes with Apples and Walnuts

Yield: 1 serving

3/4 cup to 1 cup Kashi Seven Whole Grains Flakes
3/4 cup to 1 cup low-fat milk
1/4 cup apples
1   tablespoon walnuts
1   teaspoon flaxseeds
Cinnamon to taste

In a bowl mix the cereal with the milk and cinnamon. Top with the apples and walnuts. Sprinkled the freshly grinded flaxseeds and serve immediately.

Option: Add 1 ½ scoop protein powder which adds 150 calories

Per Serving (3/4 cup Kashi and 3/4 cup low-fat milk): 303 Cal (29% from Fat, 15% from Protein, 56% from Carb); 12 g Protein; 10 g Tot Fat; 3 g Sat Fat; 2 g Mono Fat; 45 g Carb; 2 g Fiber; 16 g Sugar; 229 mg Calcium; 3 mg Iron; 189 mg Sodium; 15 mg Cholesterol
Per Serving (1 cup Kashi and 1 cup low-fat milk): 379 Cal (26% from Fat, 16% from Protein, 58% from Carb); 16 g Protein; 12 g Tot Fat; 4 g Sat Fat; 2 g Mono Fat; 58 g Carb; 2 g Fiber; 20 g Sugar; 300 mg Calcium; 5 mg Iron; 251 mg Sodium; 20 mg Cholesterol

Fennel, Leek, and Spinach Omelet

Yield: 1 serving

1/2 teaspoon canola oil
3   to 4 eggs (or 3/4 cup to 1 cup egg beaters)
1   tablespoon low-fat milk
3   to 4 ounces leeks, white part only and thinly sliced (about 1 small leek)
3   to 4 ounces fennel bulbs, thinly sliced (about 1/3 large bulb)
1/2 cup spinach, thinly sliced
1/8 teaspoon nutmeg
Salt and pepper to taste

Heat the oil in a nonstick pan over medium heat. Add the leek, fennel, and sauté until tender, about 3 minutes. Add the spinach, lightly season, and sauté another minute or two.
   Meanwhile beat the eggs in a bowl and lightly season to taste. Mix in the nutmeg and pour the mixture into a nonstick pan. Cook until the base of the omelet has set and spread over the cooked vegetables evenly. Reduce heat and continue to cook until almost completely set, about 2 to 3 minutes. Fold over in half, cook for another minute, and serve immediately.

Per Serving (3 eggs): 367 Cal (50% from Fat, 27% from Protein, 23% from Carb); 25 g Protein; 20 g Tot Fat; 6 g Sat Fat; 8 g Mono Fat; 21 g Carb; 5 g Fiber; 6 g Sugar; 217 mg Calcium; 6 mg Iron; 323 mg Sodium; 737 mg Cholesterol
Per Serving (4 eggs): 478 Cal (49% from Fat, 28% from Protein, 23% from Carb); 33 g Protein; 26 g Tot Fat; 8 g Sat Fat; 10 g Mono Fat; 28 g Carb; 6 g Fiber; 7 g Sugar; 279 mg Calcium; 8 mg Iron; 425 mg Sodium; 983 mg Cholesterol

Scrambled Eggs with Tomatoes and Onions

Yield: 1 serving

1   teaspoon olive oil
3 to 4 ounces yellow onions, chopped (about 1 medium onion)
4 to 5 ounces plum tomatoes; peeled, seeded, and chopped (about 2 medium tomatoes)
3 to 4 ounces eggplant, skin removed and diced (about 1/2 medium eggplant)
1   garlic clove, minced
1   tablespoon freshly minced basil
3 to 4 eggs (3/4 cup to 1 cup egg beaters)
Salt and pepper to taste

Heat the oil in a nonstick pan over medium heat. Add the onion and sauté until translucent. Add the chopped tomatoes, eggplant, garlic, and cook until all liquid evaporates.

Beat the eggs in a bowl with the basil and season to taste. Pour the eggs over the vegetables. Cook over medium heat, stirring and scraping constantly with a wooden spoon the bottom and sides of the pan. As soon as the eggs begin to set, remove from heat, continue to stir for a few seconds, and serve immediately.

Per Serving (3 eggs): 377 Cal (53% from Fat, 26% from Protein, 21% from Carb); 25 g Protein; 22 g Tot Fat; 6 g Sat Fat; 10 g Mono Fat; 20 g Carb; 6 g Fiber; 10 g Sugar; 139 mg Calcium; 4 mg Iron; 254 mg Sodium; 736 mg Cholesterol
Per Serving (4 eggs): 401 Cal (50% from Fat, 25% from Protein, 25% from Carb); 26 g Protein; 22 g Tot Fat; 6 g Sat Fat; 10 g Mono Fat; 26 g Carb; 7 g Fiber; 13 g Sugar; 151 mg Calcium; 4 mg Iron; 257 mg Sodium; 736 mg Cholesterol

Eggs Baked in Whole Wheat Tortilla

Yield: 1 serving

1/4 cup onion, chopped
1/4 cup fresh mushrooms, chopped
1   cup spinach
2   teaspoons grated white cheddar
3 to 4 eggs
1   whole wheat large tortilla
1   tablespoon fresh mixed herbs, chopped
Canola oil
Salt and pepper to taste

Preheat the oven to 350°F.

Preheat a steamer. Add the spinach and cook for 2 minutes. Remove from the steamer and press out any water from the spinach.

Grease a deep ovenproof dish with canola oil. Center and mold a tortilla to the dish. Top the tortilla with the onions, mushrooms, cooked spinach, and herbs. In a bowl whisk the eggs slightly, season to taste, and mix in with the vegetables. Sprinkle the cheddar cheese. Fold the tortilla over and bake for 15 to 20 minutes or until the eggs are cooked through. Transfer to a serving plate and serve immediately.

Per Serving (3 eggs): 456 Cal (45% from Fat, 26% from Protein, 29% from Carb); 29 g Protein; 23 g Tot Fat; 7 g Sat Fat; 9 g Mono Fat; 33 g Carb; 3 g Fiber; 4 g Sugar; 238 mg Calcium; 6 mg Iron; 522 mg Sodium; 742 mg Cholesterol
Per Serving (4 eggs): 541 Cal (48% from Fat, 27% from Protein, 25% from Carb); 36 g Protein; 28 g Tot Fat; 9 g Sat Fat; 11 g Mono Fat; 33 g Carb; 3 g Fiber; 4 g Sugar; 268 mg Calcium; 7 mg Iron; 603 mg Sodium; 987 mg Cholesterol

Poached Eggs over Bell Peppers and Spinach

Yield: 1 serving

3 to 4 eggs
1 teaspoon olive oil
4 ounces onions, sliced (about 1 medium onion)
1 garlic clove, minced
4 ounces red bell peppers, seeded, ribs removed, and thinly sliced (about 1 medium bell pepper)
4 ounces fresh spinach, thinly sliced
1 pinch nutmeg
Salt and pepper to taste

Grease an elongated casserole with olive oil and set aside.
Heat the oil in a nonstick pan over medium heat. Add the onion and sauté until translucent. Add the garlic, bell peppers, and cook for 2 minutes. Add the spinach, nutmeg, and season to taste.

Meanwhile bring a pan filled with water to boil. Reduce the heat under the boiling water to a point where the water barely bubbles. Break the eggs and slide them one by one into the simmering water. Make sure the eggs do not touch.

Spread the vegetables on the casserole. Using a slotted spoon carefully transfer the eggs to the prepared casserole, sprinkle pepper, and serve immediately.

Per Serving (3 eggs): 420 Cal (47% from Fat, 26% from Protein, 26% from Carb); 28 g Protein; 23 g Tot Fat; 6 g Sat Fat; 10 g Mono Fat; 28 g Carb; 7 g Fiber; 12 g Sugar; 263 mg Calcium; 7 mg Iron; 341 mg Sodium; 736 mg Cholesterol
Per Serving (4 eggs): 505 Cal (50% from Fat, 28% from Protein, 22% from Carb); 35 g Protein; 29 g Tot Fat; 8 g Sat Fat; 12 g Mono Fat; 29 g Carb; 7 g Fiber; 12 g Sugar; 294 mg Calcium; 8 mg Iron; 423 mg Sodium; 981 mg Cholesterol

Bell Peppers and Turkey Roll

Yield: 1 serving

6 ounces yellow squash, cut into strips
(about 1 medium squash)
6 ounces bell peppers, seeded, ribs removed, and cut into strips
(about 1 medium bell pepper)
2 tablespoon sun-dried tomatoes, minced
6 to 8 ounces turkey slices (about 1 ounce each or 6 to 8 slices)
6 to 8 tablespoons eggplant spread
12 to 16 basil leaves
Salt and pepper to taste

Mix the sun-dried tomatoes and eggplant spread in a bowl. Lay each turkey slice on a large cutting board. Spread 1 tablespoon of the prepared mixture and 2 basil leaves over each turkey slice. Divide equally the bell peppers and zucchini strips and season to taste. Roll up each turkey slice and serve immediately.

Per Serving (6 turkey slices): 361 Cal (31% from Fat, 34% from Protein, 34% from Carb); 34 g Protein; 14 g Tot Fat; 1 g Sat Fat; 2 g Mono Fat; 34 g Carb; 6 g Fiber; 14 g Sugar; 63 mg Calcium; 4 mg Iron; 2420 mg Sodium; 70 mg Cholesterol
Per Serving (8 turkey slices): 447 Cal (32% from Fat, 36% from Protein, 32% from Carb); 43 g Protein; 17 g Tot Fat; 1 g Sat Fat; 3 g Mono Fat; 39 g Carb; 6 g Fiber; 16 g Sugar; 70 mg Calcium; 4 mg Iron; 3208 mg Sodium; 93 mg Cholesterol

Chicken and Vegetables Roll

Yield: 1 serving

6 ounces zucchini, cut into strips (about 1 medium zucchini)
6 ounces red bell peppers, seeded, ribs removed, and cut into strips (about 1 medium bell pepper)
6 to 8 ounces chicken breast slices (about 1 ounce each or 6 to 8 slices)
6 to 8 tablespoons tapenade
Salt and pepper to taste

Lay each chicken slices on a large cutting board. Spread 1 tablespoon of tapenade over each chicken slice. Divide equally the zucchini and bell pepper strips among the chicken slices. Season to taste, roll and serve immediately or refrigerate until needed.

Per Serving (6 ounces chicken): 449 Cal (49% from Fat, 28% from Protein, 23% from Carb); 32 g Protein; 25 g Tot Fat; 3 g Sat Fat; 0 g Mono Fat; 27 g Carb; 4 g Fiber; 11 g Sugar; 51 mg Calcium; 2 mg Iron; 2649 mg Sodium; 61 mg Cholesterol
Per Serving (8 ounces chicken): 574 Cal (51% from Fat, 28% from Protein, 20% from Carb); 42 g Protein; 34 g Tot Fat; 4 g Sat Fat; 0 g Mono Fat; 30 g Carb; 4 g Fiber; 11 g Sugar; 54 mg Calcium; 2 mg Iron; 3526 mg Sodium; 82 mg Cholesterol

Grapefruit and Ahi Ceviche

Yield: 1 serving

6 to 8 ounces Ahi, Sushi grade
3 ounces onions, diced (about 1/2 medium onion)
1 jalapeno chiles, diced
1/2 cup lime juice
1/4 cup grapefruit juice
2 tablespoons cilantro, minced
1 grapefruit
Salt and pepper to taste

Mix the lime and grapefruit juices. Add the onion, jalapeno, cilantro, and season to taste. Dice the Ahi and spread it on a wide and deep glass dish. Cover the fish with the flavored juices. Mix well and refrigerate for 30 minutes to an hour.

Cut the grapefruit in half. Using a spoon, carefully move around to loosen up the flesh. Do not break the grapefruit bases, as you will use them later on in the presentation. Dice the flesh and set aside.

Mix the diced grapefruit with the ceviche. Equally divide among the grapefruit halves and serve immediately.

Per Serving (6 ounces Ahi): 448 Cal (17% from Fat, 37% from Protein, 45% from Carb); 44 g Protein; 9 g Tot Fat; 2 g Sat Fat; 3 g Mono Fat; 53 g Carb; 6 g Fiber; 35 g Sugar; 93 mg Calcium; 3 mg Iron; 74 mg Sodium; 65 mg Cholesterol
Per Serving (8 ounces Ahi): 529 Cal (19% from Fat, 42% from Protein, 39% from Carb); 57 g Protein; 12 g Tot Fat; 3 g Sat Fat; 4 g Mono Fat; 53 g Carb; 6 g Fiber; 35 g Sugar; 98 mg Calcium; 3 mg Iron; 97 mg Sodium; 86 mg Cholesterol

Fish/Seafood Entrees

A healthy diet should include plenty of fish and some shellfish, good sources of protein, fats, vitamins, and minerals, as well as many essential amino acids. In addition, one of the best sources for Omega-3 are oily fish like cod, tuna, salmon, sardines, herring, mackerel, trout, and anchovies—which are all easier to digest than meat.

You may have already heard about the health benefits of Omega-3 fatty acids, which help promote weight loss while still having a positive effect on the metabolizing of muscle proteins. Keep in mind that the protein levels of shellfish are usually a little lower than fish and, from a nutrition standpoint, can result in higher cholesterol. So be sure not to indulge on shellfish. Cooking fish and shellfish requires particular attention, as the flesh tends to be rather delicate. It is recommended that you use healthier cooking techniques such as steaming, baking, broiling, barbecuing, or sautéing in a nonstick pan with very little oil.

Shrimp with Basil and Garlic

Yield: 2 servings

2   tablespoons olive oil
12 to 16 ounces shrimps, shelled and
    deveined
2   cups onions, sliced (about 2 large onions)
2   cups bell peppers; seeded, ribs removed,
and sliced (about 4 medium bell peppers)

4   large garlic cloves, minced
1   lemon, juiced
4   tablespoons fresh basil, minced
6 to 8 ounces whole wheat pasta
Salt and pepper to taste

Cook the pasta according to package directions.
Heat 1 tablespoon of oil and the garlic in a large pan over medium heat. Add the shrimp and cook for 1 minute stirring occasionally. In another pan, heat the remaining oil. Add the onion and sauté until translucent. Add the bell pepper and sauté for another couple of minutes. Add a little lemon juice, basil, shrimp, pasta, and season to taste. Mix and continue to sauté for 1 to 2 minutes. Serve immediately.

Per Serving (6 ounces shrimp and 6 ounces cooked pasta): 747 Cal (21% from Fat, 27% from Protein, 53% from Carb); 52 g Protein; 18 g Tot Fat; 3 g Sat Fat; 11 g Mono Fat; 104 g Carb; 8 g Fiber; 11 g Sugar; 265 mg Calcium; 9 mg Iron; 275 mg Sodium; 259 mg Cholesterol
Per Serving (8 ounces shrimp and 8 ounces cooked pasta): 906 Cal (19% from Fat, 29% from Protein, 53% from Carb); 68 g Protein; 20 g Tot Fat; 3 g Sat Fat; 11 g Mono Fat; 126 g Carb; 8 g Fiber; 11 g Sugar; 306 mg Calcium; 12 mg Iron; 361 mg Sodium; 345 mg Cholesterol

Spicy Tuna with Avocado Spread

Yield: 2 servings

1   tablespoon olive oil
Two 6 to 8-ounce tuna fillets
1   large onion)
12 ounces Roma tomatoes, peeled and
    diced (about 2 large tomatoes)
12 ounces yellow bell peppers; seeded, ribs
    removed, and diced (about 2 medium
    bell peppers)

1   jalapeno, seeded and diced
1/2 avocado, puréed
2   tablespoons low-fat yogurt
1   tablespoon cilantro
1/4 lime, juiced
Tabasco
Cajun spices
Salt to taste

Mix the avocado with the lime juice. Mix in the yogurt, jalapeno chiles, cilantro, and season to taste. Add tabasco to taste and refrigerate until needed.

Preheat the broiler. Sprinkle Cajun spices on both sides of the fillets. Place the fillets on a greased baking sheet and broil for 2 to 3 minutes. Turnover and continue to cook for 3 to 4 minutes or until the fish flesh starts to flake. You may slightly salt before serving.

Meanwhile heat the remaining oil in a large pan over medium heat. Add the onion and sauté until translucent. Add the yellow bell peppers and continue to sauté for 2 minutes. Mix in the tomatoes and cook for more 2 minutes. Add a little Cajun spices and lightly salt.

Plate the vegetables, top with the tuna, avocado spread, and serve immediately.

Per Serving (6 ounces): 452 Cal (32% from Fat, 39% from Protein, 29% from Carb); 46 g Protein; 16 g Tot Fat; 3 g Sat Fat; 10 g Mono Fat; 34 g Carb; 8 g Fiber; 10 g Sugar; 115 mg Calcium; 3 mg Iron; 90 mg Sodium; 79 mg Cholesterol
Per Serving (8 ounces): 514 Cal (29% from Fat, 45% from Protein, 26% from Carb); 59 g Protein; 17 g Tot Fat; 3 g Sat Fat; 10 g Mono Fat; 34 g Carb; 8 g Fiber; 10 g Sugar; 124 mg Calcium; 3 mg Iron; 111 mg Sodium; 104 mg Cholesterol

Broiled Salmon with Pesto

Yield: 2 servings

2 tablespoons olive oil	Four 6 to 8-ounce salmon fillets
4 tablespoons basil	2 cups broccoli
2 tablespoons almonds	2 cups cherry tomatoes
1 large garlic clove	2 tablespoons Italian breadcrumbs
1 teaspoon fresh thyme	1/2 lemon cut into 2 wedges
1 teaspoon lemon zest	Salt and pepper to taste
1 teaspoon lemon juice	

In a food processor puree the basil, almonds, garlic, thyme, lemon zest, lemon juice, and olive oil. Season to taste and set aside.

Preheat the oven to 400° F. Spread the pesto over the salmon fillets and top with Italian breadcrumbs. Grease a baking sheet and add the fillets. Bake for 7 to 8 minutes or until the flesh starts to flake. Time may vary based on the thickness of the fish. Meanwhile preheat a steamer over high heat. Turn the broiler on and brown the fish breadcrumbs until golden brown, about 2 minutes. Steam the broccoli for 1 minute. Add the tomatoes and continue to steam for 1 minute. Serve the fillets with the broccoli, tomatoes, and lemon wedges.

Per Serving (6 ounces salmon fillet): 509 Cal (46% from Fat, 33% from Protein, 20% from Carb); 44 g Protein; 27 g Tot Fat; 5 g Sat Fat; 15 g Mono Fat; 26 g Carb; 7 g Fiber; 6 g Sugar; 567 mg Calcium; 4 mg Iron; 218 mg Sodium; 66 mg Cholesterol
Per Serving (8 ounces salmon fillet): 589 Cal (45% from Fat, 37% from Protein, 18% from Carb); 56 g Protein; 30 g Tot Fat; 6 g Sat Fat; 16 g Mono Fat; 26 g Carb; 7 g Fiber; 6 g Sugar; 709 mg Calcium; 5 mg Iron; 260 mg Sodium; 88 mg Cholesterol

Steamed Salmon with Fennel

Yield: 2 servings

Two 6 to 8-ounce salmon fillets	2 garlic cloves, minced
4 ounces leeks, julienned (about 1 medium leek)	2 tablespoons Pastis or anisette (you may substitute vegetable stock)
4 ounces carrots, julienned (about 1 small carrot)	2 pinches Herbs de Provence
24 ounces fennel bulbs, julienned (about 2 large bulbs)	1 teaspoon fennel seeds
	Salt and pepper to taste

Preheat the oven to 400° F.

Prepare two aluminum foil packets. Place the vegetables in the center of the foil, spread the fennel seeds, and season to taste. Top with the seasoned fish and sprinkle the Herbs de Provence. Fold the aluminum foil a bit; add the Pastis, and close tightly. Place on a baking dish and bake for 10 to 12 minutes or until the salmon starts to flake. Transfer each foil to a serving plate, open carefully, and serve immediately.

Per Serving (6 ounces salmon): 456 Cal (20% from Fat, 38% from Protein, 42% from Carb); 44 g Protein; 11 g Tot Fat; 3 g Sat Fat; 3 g Mono Fat; 49 g Carb; 14 g Fiber; 5 g Sugar; 707 mg Calcium; 6 mg Iron; 453 mg Sodium; 66 mg Cholesterol
Per Serving (8 ounces salmon): 536 Cal (23% from Fat, 41% from Protein, 36% from Carb); 56 g Protein; 14 g Tot Fat; 3 g Sat Fat; 4 g Mono Fat; 49 g Carb; 14 g Fiber; 5 g Sugar; 848 mg Calcium; 6 mg Iron; 495 mg Sodium; 88 mg Cholesterol

Cod Fish with Vegetable Slaw

Yield: 2 servings

1 teaspoon olive oil
Two 6 to 8-ounce cod fillets
2 medium Jicama
2 medium red bell peppers; seeded, ribs removed and julienned
8 ounces carrots, julienned (about 2 medium carrots)

2 green onions, julienned
4 tablespoons olive oil
4 tablespoons lime juice
4 tablespoon fresh parsley, minced
5 pinches ground cumin
Salt and pepper to taste

Place the julienned Jicama, red bell peppers, carrots, and green onions in a bowl. Whisk 4 tablespoons olive oil, lime juice, parsley, and 4 pinches ground cumin. Add the dressing to the vegetables, season to taste, mix well, and set aside.

Sprinkle pepper and ground cumin over both sides of the fish. Heat 1 teaspoon in nonstick pan over medium heat. Add the fish and sauté until golden brown, about 2 minutes. Turnover and continue to cook until the fish starts to flake.

Meanwhile quickly sauté the prepared slaw in a nonstick pan over medium heat. Lightly season the cod fillets with salt, if desired.

Transfer the slaw to two serving plates, top with the cod fillets, and serve immediately.

Per Serving (6 ounces cod fillet): 573 Cal (48% from Fat, 24% from Protein, 28% from Carb); 35 g Protein; 31 g Tot Fat; 4 g Sat Fat; 22 g Mono Fat; 41 g Carb; 16 g Fiber; 17 g Sugar; 131 mg Calcium; 4 mg Iron; 190 mg Sodium; 73 mg Cholesterol
Per Serving (8 ounces cod fillet): 620 Cal (45% from Fat, 29% from Protein, 26% from Carb); 45 g Protein; 32 g Tot Fat; 4 g Sat Fat; 22 g Mono Fat; 41 g Carb; 16 g Fiber; 17 g Sugar; 140 mg Calcium; 4 mg Iron; 221 mg Sodium; 98 mg Cholesterol

Jamaican Red Snapper

Yield: 2 servings

Two 6 to 8-ounce red snapper fillets
10 ounces carrots cut into thin diagonal slices (about 2 medium carrots)
10 ounces yellow squash cut into thin diagonal slices (about 2 medium squash)
12 ounces pea pods
2 large garlic cloves, minced

2 tablespoons fresh ginger, minced
2 teaspoons low-sodium soy sauce
4 tablespoons chives, chopped
4 teaspoons sesame oil
Jamaican jerk spices or rub
Salt and pepper to taste

Preheat a pan with water. Parboil each vegetables (carrots, squash, and pea pods) separately and until barely tender. Blanch immediately in ice cold water to stop the cooking process.

Preheat the broiler with the rack five inches away from the broiler. Spread the spices over the fillets and place them on a greased cookie sheet. Broil for a few minutes or until the fillets starts to flake. Time may vary based on thickness.

Meanwhile heat the oil in a large nonstick pan over medium heat. Sauté the ginger and garlic quickly. Add the vegetables and sauté for another minute. Add the soy sauce, chives, and season with pepper. Bring to a boil and serve immediately with the red snapper fillets.

Per Serving (6 ounces red snapper fillet): 454 Cal (24% from Fat, 39% from Protein, 37% from Carb); 45 g Protein; 13 g Tot Fat; 2 g Sat Fat; 4 g Mono Fat; 42 g Carb; 11 g Fiber; 17 g Sugar; 254 mg Calcium; 5 mg Iron; 526 mg Sodium; 63 mg Cholesterol
Per Serving (8 ounces red snapper fillet): 511 Cal (23% from Fat, 44% from Protein, 33% from Carb); 57 g Protein; 13 g Tot Fat; 2 g Sat Fat; 4 g Mono Fat; 42 g Carb; 11 g Fiber; 17 g Sugar; 272 mg Calcium; 6 mg Iron; 562 mg Sodium; 84 mg Cholesterol

Tuna Burgers

Yield: 2 servings

4 to 5 ounces potatoes, skin removed
2 to 4 tablespoons low-fat canola mayonnaise
2 to 4 teaspoons Dijon mustard
2 to 4 tablespoons basil, minced
1/2 to 1 teaspoon garlic powder
12 to 16 ounces tuna, finely chopped

Tabasco sauce
4 tomato slices
4 onion slices
4 lettuce leaves
2 buns
1 teaspoon canola oil

Peel and cook the potato in salted boiling water until very tender. Mash the potato in a large bowl. Add the mayonnaise, mustard, basil, garlic powder, and season to taste. Mix in the finely chopped tuna, add tabasco to taste, and form two thick patties. Prepare the barbecue on medium heat. Brush the tuna burgers with a little canola oil and grill for 3 to 4 minutes on each side. Slightly grill the buns on the barbecue.

Spread a little Dijon mustard on the inside of the buns. Add the tuna burgers, tomato slices, onion slices, lettuce leaves and serve immediately.

Per Serving (4 ounces potato and 6 ounces tuna fillet): 426 Cal (20% from Fat, 44% from Protein, 36% from Carb); 47 g Protein; 10 g Tot Fat; 2 g Sat Fat; 4 g Mono Fat; 38 g Carb; 5 g Fiber; 6 g Sugar; 106 mg Calcium; 4 mg Iron; 349 mg Sodium; 80 mg Cholesterol
Per Serving (5 ounces potato and 8 ounces tuna fillet): 537 Cal (22% from Fat, 45% from Protein, 33% from Carb); 61 g Protein; 13 g Tot Fat; 2 g Sat Fat; 4 g Mono Fat; 44 g Carb; 5 g Fiber; 7 g Sugar; 125 mg Calcium; 5 mg Iron; 445 mg Sodium; 109 mg Cholesterol

Snapper en Papilotte

Yield: 2 servings

2 teaspoons grapeseed oil
Two 6 to 8-ounce red snapper fillets
1 shallot, sliced
1 teaspoon lemon zest
2 tablespoons lemon juice
1 garlic clove, minced

2 teaspoons parsley, minced
2 teaspoons capers
2 cups broccoli
2 cups yellow squash
Salt and pepper to taste

Preheat the oven to 400° F.
Prepare two aluminum foil packets. Place each red snapper fillet in the middle and season lightly. Equally divide and add the lemon zest, garlic, parsley, and capers. Drizzle 1 teaspoon olive oil and 1 tablespoon lemon juice per portion. Fold the foil and place on cookie sheet. Bake for 10 to 15 minutes or until the fish starts to flake.

Meanwhile preheat a steamer. Add the broccoli, yellow squash, and steam for 2 to 3 minutes or until desired doneness. Serve immediately with the papilottes.

Per Serving (6 ounces red snapper fillet): 296 Cal (22% from Fat, 53% from Protein, 25% from Carb); 40 g Protein; 7 g Tot Fat; 1 g Sat Fat; 1 g Mono Fat; 19 g Carb; 4 g Fiber; 5 g Sugar; 148 mg Calcium; 2 mg Iron; 230 mg Sodium; 63 mg Cholesterol
Per Serving (8 ounces red snapper fillet): 353 Cal (21% from Fat, 58% from Protein, 21% from Carb); 52 g Protein; 8 g Tot Fat; 1 g Sat Fat; 1 g Mono Fat; 19 g Carb; 4 g Fiber; 5 g Sugar; 166 mg Calcium; 2 mg Iron; 267 mg Sodium; 84 mg Cholesterol

Meat / Poultry Entrees

It is important to your health that you choose a good source of protein and make sure you get the right amount. You may already know that animal protein is not as healthy for you as the protein from fresh fruits and vegetables; this is because meat can raise cholesterol levels. To minimize cholesterol, look for lean protein sources. Additionally, seek out organic meat. This is healthier for you, due to the animal's natural diet.

Here are some good general rules for selecting meat: choose venison or ostrich over beef, and choose white meat such as chicken or turkey breast over darker meat. Note that lamb and pork, which are higher in fat, should be eaten sparingly, (this is why you will find only one recipe for each in this section.) When you do eat pork, choose pork loin tender cuts and employ healthy cooking techniques, such as those described on the following pages, which will limit the addition of fat and calories during preparation while also preserving the succulent flavor of the meat.

Turkey Burgers with Whole Wheat Buns

Yield: 2 burgers

Two 6 to 8-ounce turkey burgers
3 tablespoons Italian tomato sauce
1 tablespoon Italian breadcrumbs
2 pinches oregano
2 tablespoons basil, minced
1/2 teaspoon garlic powder
2 tablespoons black olives

4 tomatoes slices
4 onions slices
A bunch of lettuce leaves
1 teaspoon canola oil
2 whole wheat buns
Salt and pepper to taste

Place the turkey burger meat in a bowl. Mix in 1 tablespoon Italian tomato sauce, breadcrumbs, oregano, basil, garlic powder, and season to taste. Form two thick patties.

Prepare the barbecue on medium heat and grease the grill. Brush the burgers with canola oil and grill for 3 to 5 minutes on each side. Heat up the buns on the barbecue.

Spread 1 tablespoon Italian tomato sauce and olives on the inside of each bun. Add the turkey burgers, tomato slices, onion slices, lettuce leaves and serve immediately.

Serve with Eggplant Mediterranean

Per Serving (6 ounces turkey burger): 404 Cal (34% from Fat, 35% from Protein, 31% from Carb); 36 g Protein; 16 g Tot Fat; 4 g Sat Fat; 7 g Mono Fat; 32 g Carb; 4 g Fiber; 7 g Sugar; 116 mg Calcium; 6 mg Iron; 1395 mg Sodium; 116 mg Cholesterol
Per Serving (8 ounces turkey burger): 475 Cal (35% from Fat, 38% from Protein, 27% from Carb); 46 g Protein; 19 g Tot Fat; 5 g Sat Fat; 8 g Mono Fat; 32 g Carb; 4 g Fiber; 7 g Sugar; 128 mg Calcium; 6 mg Iron; 1693 mg Sodium; 154 mg Cholesterol

Lamb Chops with Garlic Spread

Yield: 2 servings

3 teaspoons olive oil
Two 6 to 8-ounce loin lamb chops
2 tablespoons minced garlic
2 teaspoons parsley
2 teaspoons minced rosemary
1/2 teaspoon dry crushed red pepper
4 cups green beans
Salt and pepper to taste

Bring to a boil enough water to cover the green beans. Add 1 teaspoon of salt, the green beans, and bring to boil. Reduce heat and simmer until tender. Drain and transfer to a serving bowl. Add 1 teaspoon olive oil, season to taste, and mix well.

Mix 1 teaspoon olive oil, garlic, parsley, rosemary, and dry crushed red pepper in a bowl. Rub the garlic spread over the lamb chops.

Heat the remaining olive oil in a nonstick pan over medium heat. Add the lamb chops and cook for 3 to 4 minutes on each side or until desired doneness. Serve immediately with the prepared green beans.

Per Serving (6 ounces lamb chops): 366 Cal (37% from Fat, 42% from Protein, 20% from Carb); 39 g Protein; 15 g Tot Fat; 4 g Sat Fat; 8 g Mono Fat; 19 g Carb; 8 g Fiber; 3 g Sugar; 116 mg Calcium; 6 mg Iron; 125 mg Sodium; 109 mg Cholesterol
Per Serving (8 ounces lamb chops): 441 Cal (37% from Fat, 46% from Protein, 17% from Carb); 51 g Protein; 18 g Tot Fat; 5 g Sat Fat; 10 g Mono Fat; 19 g Carb; 8 g Fiber; 3 g Sugar; 121 mg Calcium; 7 mg Iron; 161 mg Sodium; 145 mg Cholesterol

New York Steaks with A1 Steak Sauce

Yield: 2 servings

2   teaspoons olive oil
Two 6 to 8-ounce New York steaks
1   pound onions, sliced (about 2
    large onions)
1   pound mushrooms, sliced

2   garlic cloves, minced
2   tablespoons parsley, minced
2   tablespoons A1 Steak Sauce
Salt and pepper to taste

Preheat the broiler. Brush a little olive oil over the steaks and season with pepper. Broil for 4 to 5 minutes on each side or until desired doneness. Sprinkle a little salt before serving.

Meanwhile, heat 1 teaspoon olive oil in a nonstick pan over medium heat. Add the onions and slightly browned. Add the mushrooms, garlic, and continue to cook until the mushrooms are barely tender. Add the parsley and season to taste.

Plate the vegetables in the center of a serving platter and top with the steaks. Serve with A1 Steak Sauce on the side.

Option: You may also marinade the steaks in some A1 Steak Sauce. Pat dry before grilling.

Per Serving (6 ounces New York Steak): 526 Cal (34% from Fat, 34% from Protein, 31% from Carb); 47 g Protein; 21 g Tot Fat; 7 g Sat Fat; 9 g Mono Fat; 42 g Carb; 7 g Fiber; 14 g Sugar; 127 mg Calcium; 7 mg Iron; 362 mg Sodium; 105 mg Cholesterol
Per Serving (8 ounces New York Steak): 622 Cal (36% from Fat, 37% from Protein, 27% from Carb); 58 g Protein; 26 g Tot Fat; 9 g Sat Fat; 11 g Mono Fat; 42 g Carb; 7 g Fiber; 14 g Sugar; 131 mg Calcium; 9 mg Iron; 392 mg Sodium; 141 mg Cholesterol

Beef Tenderloins with Creamy Horseradish

Yield: 2 servings

2   tablespoons olive oil
Two 6 to 8-ounce beef tenderloins
6   garlic cloves
1   tablespoon creamy-style horseradish
1   tablespoon parsley
8   ounces onions, wedged (about 1
    large onion)
8   ounces carrots, chopped (about 2
    medium carrots)

8   ounces red-skin potatoes, quartered (about 2
    medium red-skin potatoes)
8   ounces zucchini, chopped (about 2 medium
    zucchini)
1   teaspoon fresh thyme, minced
1   teaspoon fresh rosemary, minced
Salt and pepper to taste

Puree the garlic, horseradish, parsley, and 1 tablespoon olive oil in a food processor. Season to taste and set aside.

Preheat the oven to 425°F. Place the carrots and potatoes in a roasting pan. Mix in 1 tablespoon olive oil, thyme, rosemary, sprinkle pepper, and bake for 25 minutes. Add the onions, zucchini, and continue to bake for another 20 minutes. Lightly salt before serving.

Preheat the broiler. Using half of the horseradish mixture spread a thin layer on one side of the tenderloins. Broil for 5 minutes on the horseradish side. Turnover, spread the remaining horseradish spread, and broil another 5 minutes or until desired doneness. Time may vary based on thickness. Serve immediately with the roasted vegetables.

Per Serving (6 ounces beef tenderloin): 687 Cal (38% from Fat, 25% from Protein, 37% from Carb); 44 g Protein; 30 g Tot Fat; 8 g Sat Fat; 16 g Mono Fat; 64 g Carb; 10 g Fiber; 14 g Sugar; 189 mg Calcium; 8 mg Iron; 222 mg Sodium; 105 mg Cholesterol
Per Serving (8 ounces beef tenderloin): 783 Cal (39% from Fat, 28% from Protein, 33% from Carb); 56 g Protein; 35 g Tot Fat; 10 g Sat Fat; 18 g Mono Fat; 64 g Carb; 10 g Fiber; 14 g Sugar; 193 mg Calcium; 9 mg Iron; 253 mg Sodium; 141 mg Cholesterol

Chicken Breasts with Tomato Sauce

Yield: 2 servings

1 teaspoon olive oil
Two 6 to 8-ounce chicken breasts
4 small Roma tomatoes (about 1 pound)
3/4 cup pearl onions

1/4 cup dry white wine
1 pinch Italian herbs
1 tablespoon fresh basil, minced
Salt and pepper to taste

Par-boil the pearl onions for a couple of minutes. Remove the pearl onions from the water and let cool. Peel them and set aside.

Make a small X incision into the tops of the tomatoes. Heat some water over high heat and bring to boil. Blanch the tomatoes for 15 to 20 seconds. Remove and place in ice-cold water to stop the cooking process. Peel, seed, and dice the tomatoes.

Heat the oil in a large saucepan. Add the chicken and sauté until golden brown. Turnover and continue to cook for 2 minutes. Deglaze the pan with the wine and reduce a little. Add the tomatoes, pearl onions, Italian herbs, and season to taste. Reduce heat and cook for 10 minutes or until the chicken is cooked through. Add the basil and cook for another minute. Transfer to a serving platter and serve immediately.

Suggestion: Serve with wild rice and mushrooms

> **Per Serving (6 ounces chicken breast):** 304 Cal (16% from Fat, 60% from Protein, 25% from Carb); 42 g Protein; 5 g Tot Fat; 1 g Sat Fat; 2 g Mono Fat; 17 g Carb; 4 g Fiber; 10 g Sugar; 73 mg Calcium; 3 mg Iron; 126 mg Sodium; 99 mg Cholesterol
> **Per Serving (8 ounces chicken breast):** 367 Cal (15% from Fat, 65% from Protein, 20% from Carb); 56 g Protein; 6 g Tot Fat; 1 g Sat Fat; 2 g Mono Fat; 17 g Carb; 4 g Fiber; 10 g Sugar; 79 mg Calcium; 3 mg Iron; 163 mg Sodium; 132 mg Cholesterol

Chicken Breasts with Spinach and Pepper Jack

Yield: 2 servings

1 teaspoon olive oil
Two 6 to 8-ounce chicken breasts
2 Pepper Jack Cheese slices
8 spinach leaves, cleaned and pat dry
1 shallot, minced
1/4 cup chicken stock

Italian herbs
4 cups fresh spinach, cleaned and pat dry
1 lemon
Salt and pepper to taste
Twine

Place the chicken breasts between two plastic wrap sheets. Flatten with a mallet until fairly thin. Sprinkle pepper and Italian herbs. Add one slice of pepper jack cheese and the spinach leaves. Roll tightly making sure the cheese has no way out and secure with twine.

Heat the oil in a sauté pan over high heat. Add the chicken rolls, placing the folded side down first. Brown and turn over. Once browned, add the shallot, stock, a teaspoon lemon juice, a pinch of Italian herbs, and bring to boil. Reduce heat, cover, and continue to cook for 10 minutes.

Meanwhile preheat a steamer. Add the spinach and cook for a minute or until barely wilted. Serve immediately with the chicken rolls and lemon wedges.

> **Per Serving (6 ounces chicken breast):** 366 Cal (34% from Fat, 52% from Protein, 14% from Carb); 49 g Protein; 14 g Tot Fat; 7 g Sat Fat; 5 g Mono Fat; 13 g Carb; 4 g Fiber; 1 g Sugar; 327 mg Calcium; 4 mg Iron; 447 mg Sodium; 126 mg Cholesterol
> **Per Serving (8 ounces chicken breast):** 428 Cal (31% from Fat, 57% from Protein, 12% from Carb); 62 g Protein; 15 g Tot Fat; 7 g Sat Fat; 5 g Mono Fat; 13 g Carb; 4 g Fiber; 1 g Sugar; 333 mg Calcium; 5 mg Iron; 483 mg Sodium; 158 mg Cholesterol

Venison with Spicy Raspberry Sauce

Yield: 2 servings

2 teaspoons grapeseed oil
Two 6 to 8-ounce venison steaks
1 small shallot, minced
1/4 to 1/2 teaspoon black peppercorns,
    crushed (based on how spicy you like)
1 pinch dry thyme
2 tablespoons aged balsamic vinegar

1/2 cup Cabernet Sauvignon
1/2 cup raspberries
2 tablespoons demi-glace (if not available, sub-
    stitute brown sauce)
1 tablespoon freshly minced parsley
Salt and pepper to taste

Puree half the raspberries in a food processor. Pass through a sieve and set aside.
    Heat the oil in a nonstick pan over medium-high heat. Add the venison steaks and sauté until golden brown. Turnover and continue to cook for 2 to 3 minutes. Transfer the steaks to a plate and cover with aluminum foil to keep warm. Add the shallots, peppercorns, thyme, vinegar, wine, raspberry sauce, and deglaze the pan. Bring to a boil and reduce liquid by half. Add demi-glace, steaks juices, season to taste, and bring to a boil. Add the steaks, remaining raspberries, and continue to simmer for a minute. Serve immediately.

Suggestion: Serve with Green Beans and Almonds

Per Serving (6 ounces venison steak): 318 Cal (29% from Fat, 59% from Protein, 12% from Carb); 40 g Protein; 9 g Tot Fat; 2 g Sat Fat; 2 g Mono Fat; 8 g Carb; 2 g Fiber; 2 g Sugar; 32 mg Calcium; 7 mg Iron; 142 mg Sodium; 145 mg Cholesterol
Per Serving (8 ounces venison steak): 386 Cal (27% from Fat, 63% from Protein, 10% from Carb); 53 g Protein; 10 g Tot Fat; 3 g Sat Fat; 2 g Mono Fat; 8 g Carb; 2 g Fiber; 2 g Sugar; 35 mg Calcium; 9 mg Iron; 171 mg Sodium; 193 mg Cholesterol

Pasta with Turkey Sausage

Yield: 2 servings

1 teaspoon olive oil
12 to 16 ounces turkey sausages, sliced
8 ounces onions, chopped (about 1
    large onion)
8 ounces red bell peppers, chopped (about 1
    large red bell pepper)
8 ounces Roma tomatoes, quartered (about
    2 small tomatoes)

8 ounces zucchini, chopped (about 1
    large zucchini)
2 garlic cloves, minced
1/4 cup chicken stock
4 ounces whole wheat penne
2 tablespoons Parmesan cheese
1/3 cup freshly chopped basil
Salt and pepper to taste

Cook pasta according to package instructions.
    Heat the oil in a large nonstick pan over medium heat. Add the sausage slices and cook until brown on both sides. Transfer the sausage slices to a large bowl. Add the onions to the pan and sauté until slightly browned. Add the bell peppers, zucchini, garlic, and sauté until tender. Add the vegetables to the sausage bowl. Deglaze the pan with the stock and reduce by half. Add the pasta, sausage slices, vegetables, tomatoes, basil, and season to taste. Add the parmesan, toss quickly until warm, and serve immediately.

Per Serving (6 ounces turkey sausage): 660 Cal (30% from Fat, 22% from Protein, 47% from Carb); 38 g Protein; 23 g Tot Fat; 6 g Sat Fat; 9 g Mono Fat; 81 g Carb; 13 g Fiber; 18 g Sugar; 218 mg Calcium; 5 mg Iron; 1742 mg Sodium; 118 mg Cholesterol
Per Serving (8 ounces turkey sausage): 751 Cal (33% from Fat, 24% from Protein, 43% from Carb); 46 g Protein; 29 g Tot Fat; 8 g Sat Fat; 11 g Mono Fat; 83 g Carb; 13 g Fiber; 19 g Sugar; 233 mg Calcium; 6 mg Iron; 2278 mg Sodium; 155 mg Cholesterol

Pork Loin with Garlic Mashed Potatoes

Yield: 2 servings

1   teaspoon olive oil
Two 6 to 8-ounce pork loins
1   pound potatoes, peeled and chopped
    (about 3 medium potatoes)
6   garlic cloves

1/4 cup low-fat milk
1   tablespoon olive oil
1   tablespoon freshly minced parsley
Salt and pepper to taste

Preheat the broiler or barbecue.
    Place the potatoes and garlic cloves in a pan. Fill with salted water and bring to boil over high heat. Reduce heat and simmer for 20 minutes or until tender.

Meanwhile brush olive oil over the pork loins. Sprinkle with pepper and grill for 5 minutes on each side or until cooked through.

Drain and transfer the potatoes to a bowl. Mash the potatoes and garlic until almost smooth. Add the low-fat milk gradually and finish with the olive oil. Mix in the parsley and season to taste.

Transfer the loins to a serving platter, lightly season with salt, and serve immediately with the garlic mashed potatoes.

Suggestion: Serve with Wild Greens with Garlic.

Per Serving (6 ounces pork loin): 518 Cal (27% from Fat, 32% from Protein, 40% from Carb); 42 g Protein; 16 g Tot Fat; 4 g Sat Fat; 9 g Mono Fat; 52 g Carb; 4 g Fiber; 4 g Sugar; 84 mg Calcium; 3 mg Iron; 110 mg Sodium; 113 mg Cholesterol
Per Serving (8 ounces pork loin): 586 Cal (27% from Fat, 37% from Protein, 36% from Carb); 54 g Protein; 18 g Tot Fat; 4 g Sat Fat; 10 g Mono Fat; 52 g Carb; 4 g Fiber; 4 g Sugar; 87 mg Calcium; 4 mg Iron; 139 mg Sodium; 150 mg Cholesterol

Soups/Salads

Soups and salads are very versatile and can be served as an appetizer, main course, side dish, or even dessert. They're quick and healthy meal options, and can be a great way to use left-overs. In addition, salad recipes don't require much cooking knowledge, as the techniques used here are very basic.

Here are a few important things to keep in mind whenever you prepare soup or a salad. First, stay away from croutons in soups and avoid unhealthy salad dressings. Healthy dressing choices include oil and vinegar or citrus juice with fresh herbs, and apple cider vinegar can be beneficial to your health due to its cleansing and healing properties. Be careful not to overcook the vegetables you add to soup bases as they will lose their nutrients. This can be tricky because a soup's ingredients will continue to cook as long as the soup is hot, even after you've taken the soup off the stove. Try to undercook the vegetables to allow for that extra time and to preserve their nutritive values. Use dry herbs at first and finish with fresh herbs (using fresh herbs at the beginning will only be a waste of money, as the flavors will evaporate during the cooking process.) For balanced nutrition, be sure to include lean proteins, complex carbohydrates, and vegetables in your soups and salads.

Beans, Vegetables, and Avocado Salad

Yield: 3 to 5 servings

4 ounces garbanzos
4 ounces black beans
4 ounces red beans
4 ounces green beans, trimmed and
    cut into bite size
1 ounce red onions, diced (about 1/4
    small onion)
8 ounces tomatoes, diced (about 2
    small tomatoes)

1 garlic clove, minced
2 tablespoons olive oil
1/4 cup white balsamic vinegar
1 ½ tablespoons freshly minced salad herbs
1 avocado, diced
Salt and pepper to taste

In a bowl mix the garlic, oil, vinegar, and herbs.
   Cook the beans separately following the packages instructions. Generally, it takes about 30 to 45 minutes to cook these types of beans.

   Place the green beans with a little salt in a pan and bring to boil over high heat. Cook to desired doneness. Strain and place immediately in ice-cold water to stop the cooking process. Strain and pat dry.

   Place all the beans and red onions in a large bowl. Add the tomatoes and dressing. Season to taste and refrigerate for an hour. Before serving add the avocado.

Per Serving (6 ounces): 369 Cal (30% from Fat, 17% from Protein, 53% from Carb); 17 g Protein; 13 g Tot Fat; 2 g Sat Fat; 8 g Mono Fat; 51 g Carb; 17 g Fiber; 6 g Sugar; 115 mg Calcium; 5 mg Iron; 20 mg Sodium; 0 mg Cholesterol
Per Serving (8 ounces): 498 Cal (30% from Fat, 17% from Protein, 53% from Carb); 22 g Protein; 17 g Tot Fat; 2 g Sat Fat; 10 g Mono Fat; 69 g Carb; 23 g Fiber; 8 g Sugar; 155 mg Calcium; 7 mg Iron; 28 mg Sodium; 0 mg Cholesterol

Beets and Chicken Salad

Yield: 2 servings

1 pound cooked beets, trimmed and diced
8 ounces Romaine heart leaves
1/2 small onion, diced
1/4 cup walnuts
2 small apples, diced and mixed with a little lemon juice (about 8 ounces)
Two 6 to 8-ounce cooked chicken breasts, diced
2 tablespoons vinaigrette
Salt and pepper to taste

Place the beets, romaine leaves, red onion, and chicken in a large bowl. Mix in the vinaigrette and adjust seasoning. Equally divide the salad in two plates. Top with the diced apple, walnut, and serve immediately.

Per Serving (6 ounces chicken breast): 456 Cal (28% from Fat, 30% from Protein, 41% from Carb); 36 g Protein; 15 g Tot Fat; 2 g Sat Fat; 3 g Mono Fat; 50 g Carb; 12 g Fiber; 31 g Sugar; 111 mg Calcium; 4 mg Iron; 2279 mg Sodium; 61 mg Cholesterol
Per Serving (8 ounces chicken breast): 501 Cal (26% from Fat, 35% from Protein, 39% from Carb); 46 g Protein; 15 g Tot Fat; 2 g Sat Fat; 3 g Mono Fat; 51 g Carb; 12 g Fiber; 31 g Sugar; 115 mg Calcium; 4 mg Iron; 2895 mg Sodium; 82 mg Cholesterol

Beef Carpaccio with Spinach and Pistachio

Yield: 2 servings

One Rump steak 12 to 16 ounces
1   cup fresh basil
2   small garlic cloves
2   tablespoons pistachio
1/4 cup olive oil
2   cups spinach
8   ounces tomatoes, quartered (about 2 small tomatoes)
Salt and pepper to taste

Place the Rump steak in the freezer. This is important in order to be able to slice it as thinly as possible. The meat must be half frozen, not totally frozen.

Place the basil, garlic clove, pine nuts, and olive oil in a blender. Season to taste and mix until smooth. If needed, thin out with a little water.

Using a sharp knife, slice as thinly as possible the Rump steak. Place the slices overlapping each other in a serving platter. Pour the sauce over the meat and marinade refrigerated for 30 minutes.

Per Serving (6 ounces rump steak): 546 Cal (59% from Fat, 31% from Protein, 10% from Carb); 43 g Protein; 36 g Tot Fat; 6 g Sat Fat; 24 g Mono Fat; 13 g Carb; 4 g Fiber; 4 g Sugar; 142 mg Calcium; 6 mg Iron; 136 mg Sodium; 70 mg Cholesterol
Per Serving (8 ounces rump steak): 617 Cal (55% from Fat, 36% from Protein, 9% from Carb); 56 g Protein; 38 g Tot Fat; 6 g Sat Fat; 25 g Mono Fat; 13 g Carb; 4 g Fiber; 4 g Sugar; 153 mg Calcium; 7 mg Iron; 170 mg Sodium; 93 mg Cholesterol

Seared Ahi Salad

Yield: 2 servings

Two 6 to 8-ounce Ahi fillets, Sushi grade
5   ounces mixed greens
8   cherry tomatoes
8   ounces carrots, sliced diagonally (about 2 small carrots)
4   ounces daikon, sliced
4   ounces sugar snap peas
1   teaspoon sesame oil

1   teaspoon soy sauce
1   tablespoon lime juice
4   teaspoons olive oil
1   teaspoon ginger, minced
1   lime
Salt and pepper to taste

Mix the sesame oil, soy sauce, lime juice, 1 tablespoon olive oil, and ginger together in a bowl. Season with pepper.

Par-boil the carrot and sugar snap peas to desired tenderness. Transfer to an ice-cold water bath to stop the cooking process. Pat dry and set aside.

Mix the greens, carrots, daikon, and sugar snap peas in a bowl with the prepared dressing. Equally divide among two plates and refrigerate until use.

Preheat 1 teaspoon olive oil in a nonstick pan over high heat. Season the fish with pepper and light salt. Sear the fish for 2 minutes on both sides. You may sear longer, if you want the center of the fish more cooked.

Slice the fish and spread over the top of the prepared salad. Serve immediately with lime wedges.

Per Serving (6 ounces Ahi): 486 Cal (38% from Fat, 37% from Protein, 25% from Carb); 46 g Protein; 21 g Tot Fat; 4 g Sat Fat; 10 g Mono Fat; 31 g Carb; 10 g Fiber; 11 g Sugar; 113 mg Calcium; 4 mg Iron; 318 mg Sodium; 65 mg Cholesterol
Per Serving (8 ounces Ahi): 567 Cal (37% from Fat, 41% from Protein, 22% from Carb); 59 g Protein; 23 g Tot Fat; 5 g Sat Fat; 11 g Mono Fat; 31 g Carb; 10 g Fiber; 11 g Sugar; 118 mg Calcium; 5 mg Iron; 340 mg Sodium; 86 mg Cholesterol

Whole Wheat Pasta and Vegetables

Yield: 2 servings

2 ½ ounces to 4 ounces whole wheat penne
2 ounces red onions, sliced (about 1/2 small onion)
8 ounces orange bell peppers, sliced (about 1 large orange bell pepper)
8 ounces asparagus, trimmed
12 cherry tomatoes

6 ounces spinach, shredded
2 tablespoons olive oil
1 tablespoon balsamic vinegar
2 small garlic cloves, minced
2 tablespoons freshly minced basil
Salt and pepper to taste

Cook the pasta according to package directions.
Preheat a steamer. Add the asparagus and cook until desired doneness.
Mix the olive oil, balsamic vinegar, garlic, and season to taste.
Place the pasta, onions, bell peppers, asparagus, and spinach in a large bowl. Mix in the dressing, basil, and season to taste. Top with the cherry tomatoes and serve immediately.

Per Serving (2/3 cup cooked pasta): 361 Cal (35% from Fat, 13% from Protein, 52% from Carb); 13 g Protein; 15 g Tot Fat; 2 g Sat Fat; 10 g Mono Fat; 51 g Carb; 7 g Fiber; 8 g Sugar; 177 mg Calcium; 8 mg Iron; 1530 mg Sodium; 0 mg Cholesterol
Per Serving (1 cup cooked pasta): 435 Cal (29% from Fat, 14% from Protein, 57% from Carb); 16 g Protein; 15 g Tot Fat; 2 g Sat Fat; 10 g Mono Fat; 67 g Carb; 7 g Fiber; 8 g Sugar; 186 mg Calcium; 8 mg Iron; 1532 mg Sodium; 0 mg Cholesterol

Roasted Tomatoes and Shrimp Soup

Yield: 4 servings

20 ounces cooked large shrimps
2 ½ pounds large tomatoes, halved lengthwise
8 ounces red bell peppers; seeded, ribs removed, and quartered
6 ounces onions, quartered (about 1 medium onion)
4 to 5 garlic cloves

1 tablespoon olive oil
2 tablespoons freshly minced Italian herbs
1 tablespoon freshly minced basil
Salt and pepper to taste

Preheat the oven to 450° F. Place the tomatoes, bell peppers, onions, and garlic cloves on a greased baking sheet. Drizzle olive oil and mix carefully. Roast the vegetables for 40 minutes or until browned. Transfer to a food processor; add the Italian herbs and purée. Gradually add enough stock to obtain a soup consistency. Refrigerate until cold.
Serve the soup with the cooked shrimp and sprinkle the basil.

This soup can also be served hot.

Per Serving: 321 Cal (19% from Fat, 42% from Protein, 39% from Carb); 35 g Protein; 7 g Tot Fat; 1 g Sat Fat; 3 g Mono Fat; 33 g Carb; 6 g Fiber; 14 g Sugar; 182 mg Calcium; 6 mg Iron; 298 mg Sodium; 215 mg Cholesterol

Pumpkin Soup

Yield: 4 servings

1 teaspoon olive oil
2 pounds pumpkin, trimmed and chopped
8 ounces onions, chopped (about 1 large onion)
1 garlic clove, minced
4 cups vegetable stock

1 cup low-fat milk
Pumpkin pie spices to taste
4 tablespoons low-fat yogurt
4 teaspoons pumpkin seeds
Salt and pepper to taste

Peel the pumpkin and cut the flesh into medium cubes.

Heat the oil in a large pan over high heat. Add the onions and sauté until translucent. Add the pumpkin, garlic, stock, milk, spices, and bring to boil. Reduce heat, cover, and simmer for 30 minutes. Puree in a food processor using enough liquid to obtain a creamy consistency. Return to pan and season to taste. Before serving; top with the yogurt and garnish with the pumpkin seeds.

You may substitute the vegetables stock with chicken stock. If so, substitute sage for the pumpkin pie spices. This soup can be served cold or hot.

Per Serving: 209 Cal (14% from Fat, 14% from Protein, 72% from Carb); 8 g Protein; 4 g Tot Fat; 2 g Sat Fat; 1 g Mono Fat; 41 g Carb; 8 g Fiber; 18 g Sugar; 227 mg Calcium; 4 mg Iron; 183 mg Sodium; 4 mg Cholesterol

Barley Soup with Chicken

Yield: 4 servings

1 teaspoon olive oil
2 ounces barley
4 ounces onions, diced
4 ounces carrots, diced
4 ounces turnips, diced

1 bouquet garni
5 cups chicken stock
8 ounces mushrooms, diced
2 tablespoons freshly minced parsley
16 ounces cooked chicken breasts, diced

Cook the barley according to package directions. Drain and set aside.

Heat the oil in a pan over medium high heat. Add onions and sauté until translucent. Add the carrots, turnips, and sauté for 2 minutes. Add the mushrooms and sauté for a couple of minutes. Add the bouquet garni, stock, and bring to a boil. Add the drained barley, chicken, and parsley. Bring to a simmer and continue to cook for a few minutes. Adjust seasonings and serve immediately.

Per Serving: 380 Cal (18% from Fat, 42% from Protein, 40% from Carb); 40 g Protein; 8 g Tot Fat; 2 g Sat Fat; 2 g Mono Fat; 38 g Carb; 6 g Fiber; 9 g Sugar; 77 mg Calcium; 4 mg Iron; 1127 mg Sodium; 87 mg Cholesterol

Country Soup with Meatballs

Yield: 4 servings

16 turkey meatballs (about 20 ounces)
1 teaspoon olive oil
8 ounces onions, diced (about 1 large onion)
8 ounces carrots, diced (about 2
   small carrots)
2 celery stalks, diced
4 garlic cloves, minced
1 small Chinese cabbage, shredded
4 ounces green beans, cut into bite size

1 can (15 ounces) diced tomatoes
8 cups chicken stock
1 bouquet garni
1 teaspoon chili powder
1 teaspoon ground cumin
2 tablespoons fresh parsley, minced
Salt and pepper to taste

Preheat the oven to 425° F. Arrange the meatballs in a single layer on a greased baking pan. Bake for 10 to 15 minutes (may vary based on meatballs sizes).

Meanwhile heat the oil in a pan over high heat. Add the onions and sauté until translucent. Add the carrots, celery, garlic, and sauté for 2 minutes. Add the stock, chili powder, cumin, bouquet garni, green beans, and cook until the vegetables are barely tender. Add the cabbage, tomatoes, parsley, and season to taste. Simmer the soup until all the vegetables are tender. Stir in the cooked meatballs and bring the soup back to a simmer. Adjust seasonings and serve immediately.

Per Serving: 350 Cal (35% from Fat, 35% from Protein, 31% from Carb); 32 g Protein; 14 g Tot Fat; 4 g Sat Fat; 5 g Mono Fat; 28 g Carb; 7 g Fiber; 11 g Sugar; 354 mg Calcium; 6 mg Iron; 470 mg Sodium; 112 mg Cholesterol

Buffalo Chili

Yield: 4 servings

1 teaspoon canola oil
8 ounces onions, diced (about 1 large onion)
6 ounces yellow bell peppers; seeded, ribs
   removed, and diced (about 1 medium
   yellow bell pepper)
2 garlic cloves, minced
1 ½ pound ground buffalo meat
1 can (15 ounces) diced tomatoes
2 ounces tomato paste

1 ¼ cup beef stock
12 ounces cooked kidney beans or pinto beans
1 teaspoon thyme
1 teaspoon oregano
2 teaspoons cumin
2 tablespoons chili powder
1/4 teaspoon cayenne pepper
Salt to taste

Heat the oil in a deep pan over high heat. Add the meat and brown slightly. Remove the excess fat rendered by the meat. Add the onions, peppers, garlic, and mix well. Stir in the tomatoes, tomato paste, stock, herbs, and spices. Bring to a boil and reduce heat. Simmer uncovered for 20 minutes or until desired thickness. Do stir occasionally. Add the beans and bring to a simmer. Adjust seasonings and serve immediately.

Per Serving: 386 Cal (12% from Fat, 48% from Protein, 40% from Carb); 47 g Protein; 5 g Tot Fat; 1 g Sat Fat; 2 g Mono Fat; 40 g Carb; 11 g Fiber; 9 g Sugar; 117 mg Calcium; 8 mg Iron; 653 mg Sodium; 78 mg Cholesterol

Side Dishes / Desserts

Oftentimes, proteins are the focus of meals. However, you must not forget about the importance of side dishes and snacks. For one thing, their nutritional value can help complete a day's minimum requirements for vitamin and mineral intake. Once more, carefully chosen snacks and side dishes keep us from becoming bored with food. This is key, for it is often boredom that leads us to binge on poor food choices.

Side dishes should emphasize plenty of vegetables and include an appropriate amount of complex carbohydrates based on your daily activities.

Always keep the fat content low in your snacks and side dishes. Snacks should not be limited to food bars, but should instead feature fresh food sources, such as fruits, vegetables, or nuts. Good high protein snack choices also include cottage cheese and yogurt.

In the following section, you will find low-fat snack and side dish recipes that also feature the right balance of proteins and carbohydrates. This aids absorption of the nutrients and helps keep your metabolism up.

At the end of this section, you will also find several dessert options. No need to worry—although recipes like Chocolate and Hazelnut Pudding and Almond Chocolate Squares are certainly delicious, these are not your traditional, high-fat desserts. Instead, these healthy alternatives give you the freedom to treat yourself while still fulfilling the requirements for a healthy, fat-burning, and muscle-building diet.

Potatoes and Celeriac Purée

Yield: 5 to 6 servings

1 ½ pound potatoes, quartered (about 3 large potatoes)
8 ounces celeriac, quartered (about 1 medium celeriac)
3 large garlic cloves
1/2 cup low-fat sour cream

1 tablespoon olive oil
1 tablespoon freshly minced parsley
1 tablespoon freshly minced chives
Salt and pepper to taste

Place the potatoes, celery roots, and garlic in a large pan. Add enough water to cover them and add 1 teaspoon salt. Bring to boil and cook until tender, about 20 to 25 minutes. Drain and transfer to a bowl. Mash with a potato masher, add the grapeseed oil, sour cream, parsley, chives, and season to taste.

Per Serving (5 servings): 194 Cal (15% from Fat, 11% from Protein, 74% from Carb); 5 g Protein; 3 g Tot Fat; 1 g Sat Fat; 2 g Mono Fat; 37 g Carb; 4 g Fiber; 4 g Sugar; 93 mg Calcium; 1 mg Iron; 70 mg Sodium; 1 mg Cholesterol
Per Serving (6 servings): 162 Cal (15% from Fat, 11% from Protein, 74% from Carb); 4 g Protein; 3 g Tot Fat; 1 g Sat Fat; 2 g Mono Fat; 31 g Carb; 3 g Fiber; 3 g Sugar; 78 mg Calcium; 1 mg Iron; 59 mg Sodium; 1 mg Cholesterol

Roasted Sweet Potatoes with Ginger

Yield: 2 servings

2 medium sweet potatoes (about 6 to 7 ounces each)
2 teaspoons grapeseed oil
Ground ginger to taste
Ground cinnamon to taste
Salt and pepper to taste

Wash and pat dry the sweet potatoes. Prick the potatoes with a fork and microwave on high for 4 to 5 minutes. Transfer each potato to an aluminum foil, close, and let stand for another 3 to 4 minutes.
Preheat the broiler. Remove potatoes from foil, cut in half, and spread the grapeseed oil over the potato flush. Sprinkle ginger, cinnamon, and season to taste. Broil until golden brown and serve immediately.

Per Serving (7 ounces sweet potato): 194 Cal (21% from Fat, 6% from Protein, 72% from Carb); 3 g Protein; 5 g Tot Fat; 0 g Sat Fat; 1 g Mono Fat; 36 g Carb; 6 g Fiber; 8 g Sugar; 61 mg Calcium; 1 mg Iron; 26 mg Sodium; 0 mg Cholesterol

Penne with Arugula and Tomatoes

Yield: 2 servings

2/3 cup to 1 cup whole wheat penne
2 teaspoons olive oil
8 ounces mushrooms, sliced
8 ounces orange bell peppers; seeded, ribs removed, and diced
2 garlic cloves, minced
3 medium tomatoes, diced (about 16 ounces)

1/2 cup vegetable broth (low-fat and low-sodium)
2 bunches arugula, chopped
2 teaspoons parmesan cheese
2 tablespoons freshly minced basil
Salt and pepper to taste

Cook the pasta according to package directions.
Heat the oil in a nonstick pan over high heat. Add the mushrooms, garlic, and cook until golden brown. Add the bell peppers, tomatoes, and sauté quickly. Add the stock and bring to boil. Reduce heat and continue to simmer for 3 minutes. Add the arugula and cook until wilted. Mix in the cooked pasta, basil, and season to taste. Sprinkle the cheese just before serving.

Per Serving (3/4 cup cooked pasta): 313 Cal (20% from Fat, 14% from Protein, 66% from Carb); 12 g Protein; 7 g Tot Fat; 1 g Sat Fat; 4 g Mono Fat; 56 g Carb; 9 g Fiber; 10 g Sugar; 98 mg Calcium; 3 mg Iron; 257 mg Sodium; 2 mg Cholesterol
Per Serving (1 cup cooked pasta): 375 Cal (18% from Fat, 13% from Protein, 69% from Carb); 13 g Protein; 8 g Tot Fat; 1 g Sat Fat; 4 g Mono Fat; 70 g Carb; 11 g Fiber; 10 g Sugar; 99 mg Calcium; 3 mg Iron; 257 mg Sodium; 2 mg Cholesterol

Pasta with Sun-dried Tomatoes and Vegetables

Yield: 2 servings

2/3 cup to 1 cup fettuccine
2 teaspoons olive oil
4 ounces onions, sliced (about 1 small onion)
2 garlic cloves, minced
8 sun-dried tomatoes in oil
8 ounces red bell peppers; seeded, ribs removed, and sliced (1 large red bell pepper)

8 ounces zucchini, sliced (1 large zucchini)
12 ounces tomatoes, quartered (about 2 large tomatoes)
4 ounces mushrooms, sliced
4 ounces cooked artichoke hearts
2 teaspoons seeded black olives, minced
2 tablespoons freshly minced basil
Dry red peppers flakes to taste
Salt and pepper to taste

Cook the fettuccine according to package directions.
Heat the oil in a large pan over high heat. Add the onion and sauté until slightly browned. Add the bell pepper, zucchini, mushrooms, and cook until tender, about 4 minutes. Add the sun-dried tomatoes, tomatoes, artichokes heart, black olives, basil, hot red pepper flakes, and sauté for 2 minutes. Season to taste and serve immediately.

Per Serving (3/4 cup cooked fettuccine): 357 Cal (20% from Fat, 13% from Protein, 68% from Carb); 12 g Protein; 9 g Tot Fat; 1 g Sat Fat; 5 g Mono Fat; 66 g Carb; 13 g Fiber; 11 g Sugar; 112 mg Calcium; 3 mg Iron; 116 mg Sodium; 0 mg Cholesterol
Per Serving (1 cup cooked fettuccine): 419 Cal (18% from Fat, 12% from Protein, 70% from Carb); 14 g Protein; 9 g Tot Fat; 1 g Sat Fat; 5 g Mono Fat; 80 g Carb; 15 g Fiber; 11 g Sugar; 113 mg Calcium; 3 mg Iron; 117 mg Sodium; 0 mg Cholesterol

Eggplant Mediterranean

Yield: 2 servings

2 pounds eggplants, both ends trimmed
(about 4 small eggplants)
4 tablespoons olive oil
2 teaspoons cumin
2 tablespoons paprika
2 tablespoons ground ginger

2 tablespoons garlic powder
2 teaspoons coriander
1 teaspoon cayenne pepper
1/2 teaspoon ground thyme
1/2 teaspoon ground oregano
Salt

Cut eggplant slices lengthwise and arrange on baking sheet.
Mix all the spices together. On both sides of the eggplants, brush olive oil, season with salt, and sprinkle the prepared spices.

Preheat the broiler or barbecue. Broil or grill until golden brown, about 2 minutes per side.

If ground thyme and oregano are difficult to find, use regular ones and minced as small as possible.

Per Serving: 398 Cal (61% from Fat, 6% from Protein, 33% from Carb); 7 g Protein; 29 g Tot Fat; 4 g Sat Fat; 20 g Mono Fat; 35 g Carb; 19 g Fiber; 12 g Sugar; 102 mg Calcium; 5 mg Iron; 19 mg Sodium; 0 mg Cholesterol

Green Beans with Slivered Almonds

Yield: 2 servings

4 cups green beans, trimmed
4 tablespoons slivered almonds
4 teaspoons grapeseed oil
2 garlic cloves, minced
Salt and pepper to taste

Place the green beans in a pan and cover with water. Add 1 teaspoon of salt and bring to boil over high heat.
Reduce heat and simmer until al dente, about 5 to 6 minutes. Drain and set aside. Briefly heat the oil with the garlic and almonds. Add the green beans, mix well, season to taste, and serve immediately.

Per Serving: 259 Cal (49% from Fat, 12% from Protein, 39% from Carb); 8 g Protein; 16 g Tot Fat; 1 g Sat Fat; 5 g Mono Fat; 27 g Carb; 9 g Fiber; 4 g Sugar; 162 mg Calcium; 3 mg Iron; 18 mg Sodium; 0 mg Cholesterol

Asian Noodles with Cashews

Yield: 2 servings

1 teaspoon canola oil
1 garlic clove, minced
2 teaspoons ginger, minced
2 teaspoons low-sodium soy sauce
2 teaspoons rice vinegar
4 to 5 ounces Asian noodles
6 ounces carrots, sliced diagonally (about 1 large carrot)

4 green onions, sliced diagonally
2 tablespoons cashews
2 tablespoons Thai basil
1 tablespoon sesame oil
Pepper to taste
Dry red pepper flakes to taste

Cook the noodles according to package instructions.
Heat the canola oil in a wok over medium heat. Add garlic, ginger, carrots and sauté 1 minute. Add green onions and sauté briefly. Add the soy sauce, rice vinegar, peanuts, basil, red pepper flakes, and bring to boil. Add the noodles and toss to blend. Finish by adding the sesame oil, pepper to taste, and serve immediately.

Per Serving (4 ounces uncooked noodles): 402 Cal (30% from Fat, 10% from Protein, 59% from Carb); 10 g Protein; 14 g Tot Fat; 2 g Sat Fat; 6 g Mono Fat; 61 g Carb; 6 g Fiber; 6 g Sugar; 97 mg Calcium; 2 mg Iron; 1414 mg Sodium; 0 mg Cholesterol
Per Serving (5 ounces uncooked noodles): 453 Cal (27% from Fat, 10% from Protein, 62% from Carb); 12 g Protein; 14 g Tot Fat; 2 g Sat Fat; 6 g Mono Fat; 71 g Carb; 7 g Fiber; 6 g Sugar; 100 mg Calcium; 3 mg Iron; 1675 mg Sodium; 0 mg Cholesterol

Wild Greens with Garlic

Yield: 2 servings

1 tablespoon olive oil
4 cups edible greens, trimmed and chopped
2 shallots, sliced
4 garlic cloves, sliced
1 lemon, quartered
Salt and pepper to taste

Heat the oil in a wok. Add the shallots, garlic, and sauté for a minute. Add the greens and sauté until barely wilted. Season to taste and serve immediately with lemon wedges.

Per Serving: 183 Cal (33% from Fat, 11% from Protein, 56% from Carb); 6 g Protein; 8 g Tot Fat; 1 g Sat Fat; 5 g Mono Fat; 30 g Carb; 7 g Fiber; 5 g Sugar; 301 mg Calcium; 5 mg Iron; 94 mg Sodium; 0 mg Cholesterol

Brown Rice with Mushrooms

Yield: 2 servings

2   teaspoons grapeseed oil
5/8 to 4/5 cup brown rice
1 ¼ cup stock or water
4   ounces onions, diced
12 ounces mushrooms, diced
1   tablespoon chives, minced
Salt and pepper to taste

Rinse the rice well and drain. Heat 1 teaspoon oil in a pan over high heat. Add the rice and sauté for a minute. Add the stock or water and bring to boil. Cover, reduce heat, and cook until tender or about 45 minutes. Time may vary, for best results refer to package instructions.

Heat the remaining oil in a pan over high heat. Add the onion and slightly brown. Add the mushrooms and sauté until golden brown. Add the chives and season to taste. Transfer to the rice and serve immediately.

Per Serving (3/4 cup cooked brown rice): 184 Cal (19% from Fat, 13% from Protein, 68% from Carb); 6 g Protein; 4 g Tot Fat; 1 g Sat Fat; 1 g Mono Fat; 32 g Carb; 3 g Fiber; 4 g Sugar; 25 mg Calcium; 1 mg Iron; 259 mg Sodium; 1 mg Cholesterol
Per Serving (1 cup cooked brown rice): 214 Cal (17% from Fat, 12% from Protein, 71% from Carb); 7 g Protein; 4 g Tot Fat; 1 g Sat Fat; 1 g Mono Fat; 39 g Carb; 3 g Fiber; 4 g Sugar; 27 mg Calcium; 1 mg Iron; 259 mg Sodium; 1 mg Cholesterol

Vegetables with Tapenade

Yield: 2 servings

1 ½ ounces black olives, pitted
2   anchovy fillets, rinsed and pat dry
1 ½ teaspoon capers
1/2 small garlic clove
1   tablespoon olive oil

Lemon juice to taste
Pepper to taste
Vegetables such as carrots, bell peppers, cherry tomatoes, and mushrooms

In a food processor purée the olives, anchovies, capers, and garlic. Add pepper to taste. Slowly add the olive oil until you obtain a smooth paste. Add lemon juice to taste.

Per Serving (without vegetables): 104 Cal (79% from Fat, 7% from Protein, 14% from Carb); 2 g Protein; 9 g Tot Fat; 1 g Sat Fat; 7 g Mono Fat; 4 g Carb; 1 g Fiber; 0 g Sugar; 42 mg Calcium; 1 mg Iron; 397 mg Sodium; 3 mg Cholesterol

Half Red Bell Pepper Stuffed with Tuna

Yield: 1 serving

6 to 8 ounces can tuna
1/2 teaspoon paprika
2   teaspoons fine herbs
1/2 teaspoon garlic powder
1   ounce onion, diced small (about 1/4 small onion)
1.5 ounce carrot, diced small (about half a carrot)

1   ounce celery stalk, diced small (about 1 celery stalk)
2   tablespoons low-fat canola mayonnaise
6   ounces red bell pepper, cut in half, seeded and ribs removed (about 1 medium red bell pepper)
Salt and pepper to taste

Mix the tuna, paprika, fine herbs, onions, carrots, celery, and mayonnaise in a bowl. Season to taste and refrigerate for 30 minutes.

Equally divide the tuna mixture between the two halves and serve immediately.

Per Serving (6 ounces tuna): 334 Cal (21% from Fat, 51% from Protein, 29% from Carb); 43 g Protein; 8 g Tot Fat; 1 g Sat Fat; 2 g Mono Fat; 24 g Carb; 6 g Fiber; 11 g Sugar; 77 mg Calcium; 3 mg Iron; 151 mg Sodium; 83 mg Cholesterol
Per Serving (8 ounces tuna): 396 Cal (19% from Fat, 57% from Protein, 24% from Carb); 56 g Protein; 8 g Tot Fat; 2 g Sat Fat; 2 g Mono Fat; 24 g Carb; 6 g Fiber; 11 g Sugar; 86 mg Calcium; 3 mg Iron; 172 mg Sodium; 109 mg Cholesterol

Tomato, Basil, and Walnut Cup

Yield: 1 serving

4   ounces tomatoes, seeded and diced
1   tablespoon chopped walnuts
2   hard boiled eggs
1/4 teaspoon olive oil
1/8 teaspoon balsamic vinegar
2   teaspoons freshly minced basil
Salt and pepper to taste

Cut the eggs in half. Remove and disregard the egg yolks.

Mix the tomatoes, walnuts, olive oil, balsamic vinegar, and season to taste. Fill egg white halves with the tomato mixture and serve immediately.

Per Serving: 112 Cal (47% from Fat, 32% from Protein, 21% from Carb); 9 g Protein; 6 g Tot Fat; 1 g Sat Fat; 2 g Mono Fat; 6 g Carb; 2 g Fiber; 4 g Sugar; 26 mg Calcium; 1 mg Iron; 117 mg Sodium; 0 mg Cholesterol

Peanut Butter and Celery Stalk

Yield: 1 serving

2 ounces celery stalks
   (about 2 pieces)
1 tablespoon
   peanut butter

Equally spread the peanut butter among the celery stalks.

The calories are for regular peanut butter. If possible, try to find a low-sodium and reduced fat peanut butter.

Per Serving: 105 Cal (68% from Fat, 16% from Protein, 16% from Carb); 4 g Protein; 9 g Tot Fat; 2 g Sat Fat; 4 g Mono Fat; 5 g Carb; 2 g Fiber; 2 g Sugar; 30 mg Calcium; 0 mg Iron; 126 mg Sodium; 0 mg Cholesterol

Tomato and Walnut Bruschetta

Yield: 1 serving

1 slice whole wheat bread
1 tablespoon tomato sauce (your favorite)
1 tablespoon chopped walnuts
3 slices lean chicken meat (about 3 ounces)

Toast the bread slice. Spread the tomato sauce and walnuts. Top with the chicken slices and serve immediately.

Per Serving: 194 Cal (28% from Fat, 36% from Protein, 36% from Carb); 18 g Protein; 6 g Tot Fat; 1 g Sat Fat; 1 g Mono Fat; 18 g Carb; 2 g Fiber; 1 g Sugar; 26 mg Calcium; 1 mg Iron; 1157 mg Sodium; 31 mg Cholesterol

Chocolate and Hazelnut Pudding

Yield: 3 servings

1 ¼ cup low-fat milk
3 extra large egg yolks
4 tablespoons sugar
2 tablespoons cornstarch

1 teaspoon vanilla extract
3 tablespoons hazelnuts
3 tablespoons Dutch cocoa powder

Preheat the broiler. Place the hazelnuts on a baking sheet and broil until slightly browned. Remove skin by rubbing them between your hands. Chopped the hazelnuts and set aside.

Bring the milk and hazelnut pieces to boil in a saucepan. Whisk the egg yolks, sugar, cocoa, and cornstarch in a bowl until smooth. Temper the egg mixture with a little hot milk stirring with a whisk. Transfer the mixture to the remaining hot milk whisking rapidly and constantly. Heat over medium heat and bring to a boil whisking the bottom and sides of the pan to avoid scorching. The mixture will thicken in about a minute. Continue to cook and whisk until a nice shine appears, about another minute. Mix in the vanilla and divide among 3 ramekins. Place a plastic wrap over the surface of each pudding and allow cooling a bit at room temperature. Refrigerate for 2 hours and serve cold.

Per Serving: 238 Cal (32% from Fat, 16% from Protein, 52% from Carb); 10 g Protein; 9 g Tot Fat; 2 g Sat Fat; 5 g Mono Fat; 33 g Carb; 4 g Fiber; 23 g Sugar; 145 mg Calcium; 2 mg Iron; 99 mg Sodium; 8 mg Cholesterol

Pomegranate and Berries Parfait

Yield: 2 servings

1 ½ cup mixed berries
2 ounces pure Acai, no sugar added
    (1 Sambazon smoothie pack)

1 teaspoon vanilla extract
1 cup low-fat yogurt
2 tablespoons pomegranate seeds

Defrost Acai.

Mix the strawberries with vanilla extract and Acai. Marinade for 30 minutes. Spoon half of the berries into four serving parfait glasses. Top with yogurt and finish with the remaining berries. Sprinkle the pomegranate seeds and serve immediately.

Option: Add Protein Powder and/or ground flaxseeds. You may substitute cottage cheese for yogurt.

Per Serving: 148 Cal (16% from Fat, 21% from Protein, 63% from Carb); 8 g Protein; 3 g Tot Fat; 1 g Sat Fat; 1 g Mono Fat; 24 g Carb; 8 g Fiber; 14 g Sugar; 255 mg Calcium; 1 mg Iron; 87 mg Sodium; 7 mg Cholesterol

Fruits with Chocolate Sauce

Yield: 2 servings

1/4 cup strawberries
1/2 cup pineapple wedges
1/2 cup pear slices
1/2 cup apricot slices
1   kiwi, sliced
1 ½ ounce semi-sweet chocolate, shredded
1 ½ tablespoon water

Equally divide the fruits among two plates.
Melt the chocolate with water over very low heat in a double boiler. Whisk until smooth. If necessary, add a little more water. Drizzle the hot chocolate sauce over the fruits and serve immediately.

Per Serving: 197 Cal (28% from Fat, 4% from Protein, 67% from Carb); 2 g Protein; 7 g Tot Fat; 4 g Sat Fat; 2 g Mono Fat; 37 g Carb; 6 g Fiber; 28 g Sugar; 39 mg Calcium; 1 mg Iron; 5 mg Sodium; 0 mg Cholesterol

Pear and Apple Minestrone

Yield: 2 servings

5   ounces apples, brunoise (about 1 apple)
5   ounces pears, brunoise (about 1 pear)
3/4 cup jasmine green tea (or your favorite)
1 ½ teaspoon honey
1/2 teaspoon pumpkin pie spices

1   small ginger root, minced
1/2 teaspoon lemon zest
1/2 teaspoon grapeseed oil

Heat the oil in a deep saucepan over high heat. Add the apples and sauté for two minutes. Add the pears, spices, ginger, lemon zest, and sauté another minute. Add the green tea and bring to boil. Remove from heat and transfer to a serving bowl. Cool at room temperature. Refrigerate for an hour or best overnight to allow flavors to develop. Serve cold.

Per Serving: 105 Cal (10% from Fat, 2% from Protein, 88% from Carb); 1 g Protein; 1 g Tot Fat; 0 g Sat Fat; 0 g Mono Fat; 25 g Carb; 3 g Fiber; 18 g Sugar; 19 mg Calcium; 1 mg Iron; 2 mg Sodium; 0 mg Cholesterol

Almond Chocolate Square

Yield: 16 servings

1/3 cup sugar
1/3 cup maple syrup
1/4 cup grapeseed oil
1/4 cup dried prunes, pureed in a blender
    (about 12 prunes)
1 tablespoon vanilla extract
2 extra large eggs
2/3 cup almond meal

2/3 cup quick old-fashioned oats, reduced
    to a flour in a food processor or blender
1/3 cup Dutch cocoa powder
1/2 teaspoon baking powder
1/4 teaspoon salt
3 tablespoons water
Grapeseed oil

Preheat the oven to 350° F. Grease a pan (8 1/2 x 9 1/2 inch) with grapeseed oil.
    Beat the sugar, maple syrup, oil, pureed prunes, and vanilla extract. Add on 1 egg at a time, constantly mixing until well incorporated. Add the almond meal, oat flour, cacao powder, baking powder, salt, and mix until all incorporated. Mix in the water and transfer to the prepared baking dish. Bake for 20 to 25 minutes. The square is cooked when a pin inserted in the center comes out dry. Remove from the oven and let cool in the pan.

You may substitute 2 egg whites for 2 egg yolks. You may freeze portions. Defrost at room temperature or in the microwave for 15 seconds or so.

Per Serving: 136 Cal (44% from Fat, 9% from Protein, 47% from Carb); 3 g Protein; 7 g Tot Fat; 1 g Sat Fat; 2 g Mono Fat; 17 g Carb; 2 g Fiber; 10 g Sugar; 34 mg Calcium; 1 mg Iron; 64 mg Sodium; 31 mg Cholesterol

Thin Peach and Apricot Tart

Yield: 8 servings

3 ounces almond meal
2 ounces oats
3 tablespoons grapeseed oil
Pinch salt
1 tablespoon almond extract

2 to 3 tablespoons ice cold water
2 tablespoons apricot preserves
8 ounces peaches (about 2 large peaches)
8 ounces apricots (about 4 large apricots)

Preheat the oven to 475°F.
    Place the oats in a blender and reduce to a flour consistency. Place the oat and almond flours in a bowl. Add salt, oil, almond extract, and mix until crumbly. Add one tablespoon water at a time and continue until the dough is smooth and sticks together as one ball. Lay the dough on wax paper and push down with your palm to flatten a bit. Roll out the dough to a round thin form. Turn over the dough to a cookie sheet. Brush 1 tablespoon preserves all over the pie dough surface. Peel the peaches, apricots, and cut in half. Core, quarter, and slice. Starting at the edge of the dough and working inward toward the center, arrange the peach slices in overlapping circles. Finish with a circle of apricot slices in the center. Bake for 15 to 20 minutes until golden brown and slightly darker edges. Heat the remaining preserves with a little water to thin out in the microwave. Remove the tart from the oven and brush with the peach preserves. Transfer the tart to a cooling rack.

Per Serving: 177 Cal (55% from Fat, 9% from Protein, 36% from Carb); 4 g Protein; 11 g Tot Fat; 1 g Sat Fat; 1 g Mono Fat; 16 g Carb; 3 g Fiber; 8 g Sugar; 33 mg Calcium; 1 mg Iron; 5 mg Sodium; 0 mg Cholesterol

High Fiber Salad

Yield: 8 servings

2 oranges, skin removed and sliced
1 granny smith apple, skin removed and diced
1 Anjou pear, skin removed and diced
1/2 cup grapes (combination of white and red)
1 cup strawberries

1/2 cup blueberries
1/2 cup raspberries
1/2 cup blackberries
1 mango, sliced
1/2 pineapple, diced
Juice of 1 orange (or lime, lemon)

Place the fruits in a bowl. Add the orange juice and mix well. Refrigerate until use.

This is a great healthy fruit salad for a party. You may add fresh minced herbs such as rosemary, basil, or mint.

Per Serving: 127 Cal (3% from Fat, 4% from Protein, 93% from Carb); 2 g Protein; 0 g Tot Fat; 0 g Sat Fat; 0 g Mono Fat; 33g Carb; 5 g Fiber; 24 g Sugar; 46 mg Calcium; 0 mg Iron; 3 mg Sodium; 0 mg Cholesterol

Acai and Almond Milk Popsicle

Yield: 4 popsicles

3.5 ounces Pure Acai, no sugar added (Sambazon smoothie pack)
4 ounces berries
4 ounces banana (about a small banana)
4 ounces almond milk

Place all the fruits and almond milk in a blender. Purée on high speed. Divide equally among 4 popsicles maker and freeze.

Per Serving: 68 Cal (25% from Fat, 11% from Protein, 64% from Carb); 2 g Protein; 2 g Tot Fat; 0 g Sat Fat; 0 g Mono Fat; 13 g Carb; 3 g Fiber; 6 g Sugar; 35 mg Calcium; 0 mg Iron; 20 mg Sodium; 0 mg Cholesterol

Strawberries and Spinach Smoothie

Yield: 2 servings

2 cups strawberries
1 bunch fresh spinach
1 banana
1 tablespoon flaxseeds
Aged balsamic vinegar to taste (optional)
Ice cubs

P lace strawberries, spinach, and banana into a blender. Puree and mix in the aged balsamic vinegar (optional). Serve immediately.

Option: Add Protein Powder

Per Serving: 178 Cal (13% from Fat, 15% from Protein, 72% from Carb); 8 g Protein; 3 g Tot Fat; 0 g Sat Fat; 0 g Mono Fat; 37 g Carb; 10 g Fiber; 17 g Sugar; 206 mg Calcium; 6 mg Iron; 138 mg Sodium; 0 mg Cholesterol

Recipes inspired from:

THE SAINT-TROPEZ DIET
—*Apostolos Pappas, Marie-Annick Courtier*

THE PARK AVENUE DIET
—*Dr. Stuart Fisher, Marie-Annick Courtier*

THE PROFESSIONAL CHEF
—*Culinary Institute of America*

THE FLAVORS OF BON APPETIT 1998

FRENCH CLASSICS
—*Richard Grausman*